HEALTH CARE GONE WRONG

HEALTH CARE GONE WRONG

How Decades of Greed and Misguided Legislation Hijacked the Medical Profession

*For Everill
with love,
Phij*

Philip R. Hirsh Jr., MD

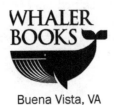

WHALER BOOKS

Buena Vista, VA

1 3 5 7 9 10 8 6 4 2

Library of Congress Control Number: 2021918378

Health Care Gone Wrong
Philip R. Hirsh Jr., MD

p. cm.
1. Biography & Autobiography: Medical
2. Medical: Physicians
3. Medical: History

I. Hirsh, Philip, 1938– II. Title.
ISBN 13: 978-1-7349136-9-9 (softcover : alk. paper)
ISBN 13: 978-1-7378864-0-2 (ebook)

Design and Layout by Karen Bowen

Whaler Books
An imprint of
Mariner Media, Inc.
131 West 21st Street
Buena Vista, VA 24416
Tel: 540-264-0021
www.marinermedia.com

Printed in the United States of America

This book is printed on acid-free paper meeting the
requirements of the American Standard for Permanence of Paper
for Printed Library Materials.

DEDICATED TO GRACE

CONTENTS

PREFACE

THE IDEA BEHIND THE FIRST completed draft of this book, titled *Remembering Grace*, was to show that our ability to efficiently deliver high quality health care has not kept pace with advances in medical technology; in fact, the reverse is true, and we are now ranked at the bottom of the world's top industrialized nations in quality, efficiency, access to care, and outcomes. The only place we take a first is in money spent to support the system. Using my own professional experience to frame the discussion and provide historical context, I focused most of the story on medical training and practice from the 1950s to roughly 1970—the point erosion began as insurance companies, the pharmaceutical industry, and legislative forces all started to muscle their way into traditional health care. The rest of the story shows how tradition and the imagined goodness of the marketplace are no match for the power of profit and bureaucratic rulemaking.

While prescient, the subject is hardly exciting; frankly, it's downright dull. I imagined animating it with first-hand true stories and observations, many funny, some scary, and others downright unbelievable. It starts with my early ambivalence about trying to go to medical school at all, doubts that diluted my college preparation, putting acceptance somewhere between farfetched and maybe. Once in, there was the shock of terror teaching, long banished from the radically different tone of today's brand of teaching. Next came internship, a murder, some other mishaps, then residency, and two bizarre years in the Army Medical Corps at the height of the Vietnam War. From there, the narrative moves quickly through the years up to today, when corporate and political interests manipulate the discussion, inhibiting rational debate on a clear path to the quality health we need and can afford.

The idea didn't work. When the draft went out to readers for comment, there was a dreadful silence. One reader didn't say anything, and a couple of others offered noncommittal variations of "Nicely written but…"

Then there were my two favorites, and the moment when it all came into focus. The first one described the book as simply, "quaint." The second, a bit more playful, but to the point, said it should be retitled, *Flashman Does Medical School.*

The *Flashman* books were about a fictional Victorian cad, an unwilling soldier and scoundrel who always managed to emerge the hero from an endless series of exploitations and narrow escapes. The books were funny and historically interesting; strangely, in spite of his miserable character, one always rooted for Sir Harry Flashman. I understood the reference, took it as a compliment, a suggestion that my near-misses and stories by themselves did have value, at least for humor.

The "quaint" reference runs a little deeper, suggesting something both pleasing and old fashioned, a connection to history. After some thought and discussion, it dawned on me that I had made an elementary writer's mistake: I assumed everyone would enjoy the historical material. Wrong. Today's reader doesn't care a bit about history. Ask someone my age (82) about the height difference between George Washington and James Madison, and there's a good chance the response would be Washington was nearly a foot taller than Madison. A younger person, asked the same question, would shrug, turn to his cell phone and say, "I'll look it up. Ah! Ten inches." We couldn't just "look it up" on the spot, so we *learned* it. But "ten inches" is certainly a better answer. A draw.

Because history isn't all that interesting to today's reader, the stories that support it would be equally ho-hum. When it comes to the debate on health care, chances are few of finding someone whose mind isn't already made up. Even if it isn't, reading sixty-year-old tales about researchers stealing livers from people who died in ERs doesn't mean much either.

To sum up: I had the history and stories right, but misjudged the audience. Far more anecdotal than academic, this is really a book of short stories and observations mourning the loss of honor, art, and the joy of practicing quality medicine.

Why be so blunt about my shortcomings? Because I think the lessons I learned are worth some thought by themselves. Plus, I want to be honest about whom I think would most likely enjoy these tales.

If you are standing in front of the book rack reading this to see if you want to read more, and you are an older reader with a sense of humor, possibly with an interest in medicine, and open to at least considering my suggestions, then you might enjoy *Health Care Gone Wrong*. If you are holding the book in one hand, a cell phone in the other, and aren't particularly interested in the gory details of medical training and practice sixty years ago, you should probably put it back in the rack. ← *what a way to begin*

1

THE RABBIT HOLE

"You are old, Father William," the young man said,
"And your hair has become very white.
Yet you incessantly stand on your head—
Do you think at your age it is right?"
(Lewis Carroll; *Alice's Adventures in Wonderland*)

POOR FATHER WILLIAM, DISMISSED BEFORE he could speak, his accumulated wisdom of no interest to an audience whose only curiosity was how he was able to balance an eel on the end of his nose.

Carroll had his eye on a timeless problem we old goats face when talking about what we have learned and may want to pass on to others. Tell the story about the time Grandmother drove her golf cart into the duck pond and they're right with you. But they glaze over the instant you start in on how it used to be back when candy bars cost a nickel.

Aware of the twin perils of pedantry and nostalgia, and using plenty of golf cart stories, I want to take you on a politically incorrect tour of physician training a half century ago, tracing a causal pathway through the evolution (or perhaps, "devolution") of medical training and practice from the 1950s to today. Knowing the past informs the present, and given the enormous debate swirling around health care today, a little perspective may add some depth to the discussion. A little humor won't hurt, either.

Most of the story is focused between the mid-1950s and 1970, the time it took me to transition from college to medical school, through internship, residency, and two years in the Army during the Vietnam War. I started practice in 1970 and will limit the narrative at that point to avoid shifting the focus away from being an observer-reporter to a personal report on my practice. Talking about practice would inevitably mean talking about individual patients, an inviolable realm of confidentiality.

don't think I know this!

While I don't want to drift too far off course into a discussion of the political and economic issues that shaped health care over the years, a brief overview of some of the game changing forces will better frame the story.

In the time since I started training, control of health care practice has transformed from a laissez-faire group of individual practitioners to a highly regulated, profit-focused system in which physicians are simply pawns in the scheme. Private practice is gone, replaced by employment in corporate health systems. Entire practices have been bought to feed corporately owned hospitals, and office managers dictate practice expectations down to a granular level, starting with the expectation a physician will see 16–18 cases a day, no matter their complexity.

Reacting to that last fact, one medical school dean said, "We've adopted the HMO business model. Office managers match time spent with patients to revenue produced. You simply can't be a good doctor averaging twelve minutes per patient."

Following the corporate model, physicians are now "providers," along with nurses and everyone else in the system. Because their salaries are carefully metered, and mediocre compared to a few other specialties, newly minted physicians avoid family practice, heading instead where the money is.

The transition is the result of the interplay of convoluted legislation and free market manipulation, starting with the earth-shaking introduction of Medicare and Medicaid in 1965.

The battle against some form of government-supported health care started in the late 1930s, intensified in the 1950s, and reached a fevered pitch before a system channeling the cost of elder health care through Social Security became law. To some it was radical, to others it was timid. In reality, Medicare was initially quite modest in scope, and Medicaid only impacted a relatively small number of "welfare" patients.

When I finished training in 1970, health insurance was more help than hindrance. In a 1971 newsletter, Blue Cross Blue Shield in Washington, DC, even *bragged* about adding psychiatric outpatient care to its benefits package. They had discovered that patients receiving mental health treatment filed significantly fewer other health-related claims, data showing the multiple benefits and cost effectiveness of meaningful psychotherapy.

How quickly things change! Within a few years, claims for therapy swamped the Blues, so they reversed field and started throwing up barriers to treatment.

By the mid-1970s, self-pay for care had shifted dramatically to reliance on health insurance, pushing the insurance companies to tighten their criteria for compensation in order to maintain profits. They found they could better protect the vault by boldly intruding into the realm of medical decision-making, previously the exclusive purview of physicians. They could get away with it because of a 1974 law, the Federal Employee Retirement Income Security Act, or "ERISA," originally designed to protect employee benefit and retirement accounts, like your 401K plan, plus give wronged consumers access to remedy.

But legislating good ideas is often a bad idea, especially when special interests twist simplicity into ambiguity on the way to getting courts to undermine protections. In the ERISA case, it went full circle, becoming a tool to preempt state law so people can't easily sue an insurance company for decisions it forces upon physicians and patients.

A New York judge said of ERISA: It "ranks high in law's order of absurdity." The Supreme Court upheld the law in 1987, and it still holds today, surviving attacks and conflicting decisions.

In the early 1980s, the insurance industry upped the ante with the introduction of "managed care," a more aggressive form of decision-making. Like having Lilly Tomlin explain your phone bill, a double-speak vocabulary sprang up featuring a host of new words and acronyms. EOB (Explanation of Benefits) really meant "Explanation of Restrictions." "Usual and Customary Charges" translated to arbitrarily discounted fees. Denied charges said not to be "medically necessary" simply meant, "Naah, we're not paying for it." "Preexisting Condition" was a tool to deny payment for something the patient actually or even theoretically brought to the game before coverage began. That was a particularly easy ploy in the denial war because so many conditions either have or theoretically could have antecedents ahead of an acute episode. Either rationalization led to the same place: "Sorry, you're not covered."

More recently, denials have been based on an even more strangled version of "preexisting," one that doesn't even have to connect one's current illness with an antecedent disorder. In this twist, an insurance reviewer, looking back through a patient's medical record, may find the person was treated years before for some totally innocuous problem like a yeast infection or eczema. Then the individual's application form is reviewed and if that trivial, long-forgotten event wasn't listed as a previous event, even though not remotely connected to any current illness, the omission is labeled deceptive, meaning the application was invalid, and the claim is denied.

Non-medical reasons are another pathway to denial. One of the trickiest is failure by either the physician or the patient to get "Prior Authorization" from the insurance company for a particular procedure. Worse, there is no predictability to what is or is not a covered procedure. How many times has your physician given you a clear yes or no to the question of coverage for a recommended procedure? Call the insurance company is the answer. But even then, the answer may not be clear. A "yes" can turn into a rejection after the fact, and your "But I was told…" objection is countered by reference to a "Don't count on what we say" statement buried somewhere in the fine print.

Like patients who have dueled with unyielding reviewers, you will not find a physician today who doesn't have a fist full of denial stories. I have dozens, and have heard many more from colleagues, stories like the one a surgeon recently told me about a patient he had seen in an emergency room with severe abdominal pain. It was quickly realized she had an Ectopic Pregnancy; that is, a fertilized egg was lodged in the fallopian tube connecting ovary and uterus. Growth there produces excruciating pain, and unless dealt with promptly, could be fatal.

The surgeon was told he had to get authorization from the insurance carrier to operate, but to his horror, the request was denied.

"The guy sounded like he barely had a high school education, and certainly no understanding of the urgent nature of the problem." It took needless time to get it straightened out, time for more pain, and increasing danger of rupturing the fallopian tube.

Another trap is rejection of a physician's "Individual Treatment Plan" (ITP). Just when and how prior approval and/or an ITP *is* needed trips up patients and physicians alike. Also, insurance companies only accept calls or written application from the physician, not nurses or medical records personnel. More steps, more time, more opportunity to fail the process, any part ending with delayed or denied service.

The treatment plan requirement is usually required when treatment involves several steps. It applies to both outpatient and hospital care. Even the language used has to conform. For example, each step has to be written using "Observable and Measurable" markers leading to speedy resolution. On the surface, it sounds reasonable: tell us the plan so we can be sure you're not winging it or dragging your expensive feet. You can't trust doctors to do what they're trained to do. No matter how routine or standard the treatment, the process demands a unique plan (no boilerplate or repeating plans allowed) written in precise language including an exact timeline in spite of the reality that not everyone responds as anticipated or without complications. Too bad: denied. Extensions are tough to get as well. In reality, the process adds another expensive layer of unneeded documentation while adding nothing to the quality of care.

Pay attention to the word "individual" in the "Individual Treatment Plan." If in describing your plan to treat Joe's asthma the reviewer detects any hint of "boilerplate" or language failing to distinguish Joe's asthma from Bob's, then it is cause for denial. It leads to a huge waste of time trying to come up with unique ways to say the same thing, not to justify treatment or its cost, but to soothe a reviewer into approving the plan. Surgeons also face the "no boilerplate" trap. Their post-operative report must be unique, completely individual, no matter how routine the procedure.

The spillover applies to any related medical procedure covered by insurance. Take Physical Therapy (PT), for example. You don't have the slightest chance of reimbursement if you refer yourself for PT, no matter how clearly the treatment is needed, or has helped in the past. Not only do you have to go through a referring physician, often adding a needless appointment, but the physical therapist must then perform a detailed exam and complete a precise treatment plan written with "observable and measurable" treatment steps leading to resolution of the *one* specific problem. If accepted, a certain number of sessions will be allowed, each requiring a review of progress toward resolution. If more time is needed, it has to be approved. Any deviation will result in the whole program being denied.

Beyond mandated coverage for immunizations, insurance companies are reluctant to pay for prevention services. Even today after mammography and endoscopy battles seem to have been won, a discussion of nutrition, exercise, or health management, no matter how serious the primary medical condition, will not be covered. That job—if it is done at all—falls to an assistant whose labors are not billable.

Another tactic has been to require physicians—not their assistants—to call or write challenges to denials or demands for more information. That nightmare takes one straightaway into frustrating encounters with shadowy telephone "reviewers." But first, you have to outlast recorded messages and holds with endless loops of rancid music interrupted only by an oozy voice telling you how terribly important your call is. Reviewers are alleged to be nurses, putting a fig leaf over the fact that whatever their *bona fides*, they are workers paid by the insurance company to filter and pass judgment on rejection review. Of course, one can appeal. For physicians drawn into the process, it can mean the chance to talk to a physician. Finally! A colleague! Someone who understands the issues from a medical point of view! Sorry, but the results are frequently the same. His paycheck comes from the same bank as the first reviewer's check.

Physicians working in hospitals have to answer to in-house reviewers, usually a nurse specialist acting as an interface between the physician, hospital, and insurance carrier. When a physician is told the carrier will not pay for anything after a certain time—down to a specific hour—and the physician calls the carrier to beg for an extension, the standard condescending answer is: "Oh, please, Doctor! We are not *telling* you to discharge the patient. That is *your* decision." Trouble is, for a hospitalized patient, refusal really is a discharge notice because any subsequent charges fall to the patient. In the highly likely chance that the patient can't immediately pay up, by law the hospital has to go full force after the patient.

By Medicare rules, hospitals participating in Medicare are not allowed to charge a patient a fee less than what Medicare would allow. So, discounts or forgiving part or all of a fee is illegal unless the provider "opts out" of Medicare completely; once out, the provider can't get back in for two years. Similarly, forgiving a fee by simply not trying to collect it is illegal. A specified series of attempts to collect must be documented, no matter how hopeless or cruel it may seem. The same rules apply in any office practice accepting Medicare, no exceptions. Hospitals and physicians alike are forced to wring the money out of the patient. The results are often disastrous, not just in an immediate financial sense, but all too often ending with a downgrade in the patient's credit rating.

The process can also hurt the physician who has put the needs of the patient above the intransigence of the insurance carrier. How long do you think the board of that hospital will want you on its staff when you start to act in a principled way and stack up a pile of unpaid extensions?

The carriers also know that premature discharge can lead to readmission. You would think that would be a deterrent, but it is not. They calculate the number of readmits against the cost of extensions. Figuring that not all such patients will be readmitted, they have found it is cheaper to deny extensions and pay for some readmissions. Besides, if the patient goes south because of the premature discharge, the company is in the clear—it's the physician who gets sued.

In the mid-1980s, I was practicing in a hospital, finding it increasingly difficult to keep patients long enough to provide quality care. Too much valuable time was lost in lengthy and distracting meetings whose only purpose was to craft treatment plans that could justify more time. To better understand the process, I attended a large managed care conference, foolishly thinking my concerns would be addressed, and a reasonable way forward would become clear. Instead, I was stunned by the blatantly self-serving nature of managed care thinking.

One presenter, talking about reimbursement for psychiatric treatment, laid it out in unequivocal terms, saying that all previous systems were being replaced by a new, streamlined model, one he grandly proclaimed would actually *improve* treatment outcomes. His reasoning had nothing to do with science; no, it was based entirely on the notion that saving money would magically mean treatment for more people! It didn't happen, of course, because the "savings" went into company profits, not back to patients.

The justification of the new psychiatric model was based on three perceived flaws in the then-current system, starting with cost. Because any treatment—outpatient or inpatient—beyond the carrier's set limit was seen as "open-ended," it put pressure on both the patient and physician to end treatment, similar to the Physical Therapy example above. There is some truth in the argument, but it wasn't worth talking about because of the second conclusion: no matter what the cost or length of treatment, all forms of psychotherapy simply don't work at all. For inpatients, the argument was that unless suicide was an immediate issue, care could just as effectively be delivered as an out-patient.

The ineffectiveness argument was immediately challenged by several psychiatrists in the audience, citing a then-current analysis of 250 published studies showing the effectiveness of psycho-therapy, as well as its known secondary benefits to physical health.

The presenter was undaunted. He said the company had its own studies and moved on to his last point: the scope of all types of therapy is too wide, covers too much ground, and should be limited to a single presenting problem, and nothing else.

Applied to out-patient care, the new paradigm, with an approved treatment plan, usually authorized between six and ten sessions, all to be focused on one and only one problem. If more sessions were needed, an extension could sometimes be negotiated. The same principle applied to inpatient care: once approved for admission, and followed by an acceptable treatment plan, a certain number of days would be allowed to be followed by immediate discharge.

But here's the kicker: when asked how a reviewer could justify cutting off treatment in either setting, the speaker's answer was *blame the patient.* Reaching the end of the allotted time without meeting the established goals *proved the patient was resistant to care*, not ready for change, and adding more time was a waste of resources. And what happens next? After all, the patient's prob-lems would predictably continue, again become overwhelming, forcing a return for more treatment.

The answer to that one was that the patient *might not* return, but if he did, the process would simply start over. With a new approved plan in hand, six more sessions could be authorized. Bottom line: from a cost point of view, interrupted care was cheaper than fin-ishing the job in the first place. That is not my interpretation or an implied conclusion; it was stated out loud in clear words, even to the point of labeling the concept "Interrupted Care."

Another speaker urged the increased use of drugs, not just in psychiatry but across the board. Insurance companies will insist a drug regimen be tried before some procedures, no matter the consequences of their tactics, and if a trial with drug X fails, then you must try Y before doing the endoscopy to define and treat the patient's esophageal cancer masquerading as intractable heartburn.

You would think that dealing with a problem and resolving it quickly would be a cost-effective goal. But like the readmission rationalization, prevention and treatment are always secondary to profit.

Over time, psychiatric care has increasingly become a medication game, largely because of economic factors. Until the early 1970s, psychotherapy was the exclusive property of psychiatrists, but as both the popularity and cost of therapy started to rise, psychologists became more assertive, swapping their Rorschach charts for office practice. They charged less money, offered a faster treatment model, and seemed less remote and hidebound than psychiatrists. Patients and insurers alike took notice—and so did social workers. If the PhD psychologists could provide therapy, so could they—at an even better price. So began an opening up of the entire field of psychotherapy, not only in who was doing the work, but also in *what kind* of therapy was being deployed. "Psychotherapy" morphed into "Therapy," a generic term covering every form of talking treatment from Aroma to Zeitgeist, though only a fraction qualified for insurance coverage.

Psychoanalysis was out, brief therapy was in. By the 1980s, many forms of therapy had come and gone, but Cognitive Behavioral Therapy (CBT) remained an effective, learnable, cost-effective method insurance companies were willing to cover.

Coupled with more medications coming to market, psychiatrists began to move to the medication management model, initially coupled with brief psychotherapy. Inevitably, pressure on compensated time pushed "med management" into the marketplace as the remaining safe zone for psychiatrists to practice.

It wasn't just psychiatry being reshaped by market forces. Across the range of traditional practice, changes in compensation produced dramatic shifts in the way most specialties were organized. For example, in Gastroenterology (focused on disorders of the digestion track from stem to stern), office consultation was devalued while procedures like endoscopy (looking into the esophagus, stomach, and colon) were valued. Formerly, those procedures were done on referral by surgeons, but GI physicians realized they could keep the business for themselves, suddenly turning quiet offices into mini hospitals.

Carriers reacted to the greater number of procedures being performed by chipping away at compensation, starting with lowering the imaginary "Usual and Customary" fee. Take, for example, a recent colonoscopy bill for a routine procedure resulting in removal of one small polyp. The gastroenterologist billed $999 for his service; Medicare discounted it to $387 and paid $225. The anesthesiologist didn't do as well. She billed $2,000; Medicare discounted it to $133, and paid $104. The facility billed $888; that was discounted to $475, and paid $372. A total of $3,887 was discounted to $995, yielding $701—just 18% of what was billed. It is absurd on both ends, with each side in an unbridled battle to control the other.

Ophthalmologists felt the squeeze between higher costs, compensation for office care to keep up, and optometrists expanding their vision checkup and prescribing business. But advances in cataract and other eye surgeries provided a lucrative alternative path. But that, too, faced discounted carrier compensation, so like other increasingly discounted procedures feeling the pressure, maintaining income has become dependent on running increasing numbers through the mill.

Internal Medicine and family practices faced the same pressure from poor compensation, but without compensatory specialty procedures to beef up income. One Primary Care Physician (PCP) recounts receiving more insurance compensation for removing an infected fingernail in ten minutes than she did from seeing eight other patients over the next two hours. Ironically, those eight probably had more at stake than the patient with the paronychia (infected nail).

Policy changes generated through Medicare have repeatedly been proposed to help PCPs, some tried with considerable fanfare, but all have failed to deliver relief for physicians whose work is at the heart of all health care delivery. Another irony: they are the ones whose referrals feed the other specialties, and provide the documentation platform needed for them to collect their fees.

PCPs also get it from both sides in the Pharma pinch. When a drug plan turns down a prescribed drug, or the copay is beyond reach, the PCP is pulled back in to find a substitute, one that may be covered and affordable. That takes time for secretaries, nurses, and physicians, all of it hopelessly beyond any sense of being a billable service.

Time is not billable, *procedures* are. Get it?

Pressure to prescribe flows in large measure from the need to shortcut time. Cut the gab, grab the pad. That isn't to say medication is prescribed recklessly; it's more subtle than that. But too often—and not just in psychiatry—financial pressure pushes the use of drugs whose side effects can swamp any benefit. A friend reports going on referral to a rheumatologist to be evaluated for hand pain. Without even touching him, the physician said, "It's arthritis, try this," adding as an afterthought, "If this doesn't work, call us. We'll try something else."

Insurance companies always insist on the cheapest drugs first, and if an expensive one is approved at all, the lion's share of the cost will be shouldered by the patient as a co-payment. I'll have more to say about that problem in a later chapter.

No matter the specialty, insurance carriers always stand between you and your prescription. Because generic drugs are usually, but certainly not always, cheaper, the insurance company will insist on a generic first, a strategy called "First Fail." You are expected to take it until it is clearly not working before being allowed to switch.

Cost is everything; besides, insurance carriers insist there is total equivalence between trade and generic medication, a deceptive assurance. It is true that, overall, generics are as effective and safe as their trade counterparts. They must contain the same *active* compound, work the same way, and have the same effect as the trade drug. But they are not identical. By FDA rules, the *inactive* ingredients only have to be "Acceptable." For some patients there is a small risk of allergy to any new ingredient, including the dye used to color the pill.

It gets trickier. When the trade drug's patent runs out, there is no requirement that either the method of making the compound or the mechanism for releasing it has to be revealed. Generic companies must invent their own systems, and the rules allow the concentration of a product in the patient's system to differ by up to 10%, though variation is rarely more than 2–3%. Also, because absorption may be different, the timing of the drug's availability to cells may differ slightly from its trade counterpart; however, for some patients, even a slight difference can be a problem. This is particularly important for anti-seizure drugs, the blood thinner warfarin, and lithium, drugs that require a precise blood level to be both effective and safe.

At the same time insurance companies were redefining health care, the pharmaceutical industry accelerated its brand of control through aggressive pricing, physician bribery, and lobbying for legislative profit protection. The legislative part became rooted in law through the Medicare Prescription Drug Act of 2003, now widely known as Part D, one of the four major pillars of the Medicare system, along with Part A (hospital costs), Part B (doctor fees), and Part C (specific plans run through Medicare).

Most of the plan was written by Pharma lobbyists, minimally debated, and passed by a narrow margin in a flurry of last-minute vote changes based on who-knows-what kind of deals and promises.

Two particularly bizarre rules were enshrined in Part D law. First, the act prohibited insurance plans from negotiating with drug companies for discounted prices. Congress kindly extended that luxurious protection in the Affordable Care Act ("Obamacare"), making a mockery of the word "affordable." Incidentally, the Veteran's Administration is not bound by the non-negotiating rule, allowing Veterans to get medication at a fraction of the cost the same drugs cost through Part D.

The second Part D twister was the famous "Donut Hole," a bit of accounting slight-of-hand responsible for many patients suddenly being ripped off their medication until they paid an $1,800 ransom: the full, bloated price Pharma gave their products.

Here's how it worked. The patient and the plan were responsible for paying the first $2,400 of the cost of medication. Then one fell into the Donut Hole, meaning the patient became responsible for the next $1,800 out of pocket before the plan magically reappeared to pick up 100% from there on.

"What's the big deal?" you might reasonably ask. One would have to pay a zillion copays to get to $2,400; *I'm safe from the vortex*. But note, the act calculated the Donut Hole *not* just on the sum of copays, but also on what the *plan had to pay*. Let's say you take Drug X, and it is covered by your Part D plan. Pharma pegs the cost at $400 a month and your copay is $65. In Donut Land, the entire $465 counts toward the Donut Hole, not just the part you paid. In six months, you're in the ditch.

Oh, and one more twist: who gets to say how much the drug costs? Why not $300 or even $50—the price they charge in Canada for the same drug? Pharma, again. Insulated from the horror of the tiniest discount or pricing oversight, they can peg the price of each drug to the max.

Part D modifications have changed the price of donuts; mine is currently pegged at $3,500. Does the increase keep my feet out of the rising tide? Nope. Pharma simply upped the drug price to make up for the change. It's easy when you own the players who make the rules.

I have seen many sick patients suddenly and without warning tumble into the hole. Drug prices can—and do—change frequently and without warning. Even the most obsessive patients find it difficult to anticipate the edge of the pharmaceutical black hole. To keep track of where you are, you need to get the cumulative pricing information from the pharmacist with every prescription, or if you get an EOB from the Part D carrier, don't toss it! Look through it carefully until you find the calculations telling how far you have to go before Pharma-gravity pulls you into the hole.

When a patient falls over the edge and is unable to afford a certain drug, the search begins to find a generic, assuming there is one and it is affordable. Some generics are horrendously expensive, well beyond the reach of many patients. Also, moving from a trade drug to a generic is not always easy. Remember, that while the active ingredient is the same in both, slight differences in absorption, time when the drug peaks in the bloodstream, plus new allergy exposure to different inactive ingredients are all suddenly in play. This is not simply theoretical—something remote that *might* happen. Over the years, I have seen a significant number of patients struggle when switched to a generic.

Obamacare moderated but did not correct the problem. Congress showed the usual lack of backbone needed to stand up to Pharma and insurance company lobbyists. To make sure nothing gets in the way of doing business their way, they lavish over $300 million a year on their lobbyists, meanwhile paying their executives obscene, multi-million-dollar compensation packages. Pharma alone spends around $30 billion a year to market its products. When challenged over drug prices, they trot out the argument that they need the money for research. No profits, no new drugs.

But how can it be so much more expensive here than in other countries, even ones with nearly comparable incomes? The arguments are many, starting with the fact that innovation costs big bucks, money returned only through drug sales. Also, other countries take advantage of our inventiveness, coupling it with zealous price controls. None of this is as black and white as the reductionists on any side of the debate claim.

The debate over health care is on fire as I write, so the fate of the Donut Hole, drug pricing, and a host of other pivotal issues is uncertain. Who knows? Maybe Obamacare will be scotched wholesale and the Donut Hole will open its jaws even wider for new victims.

Even beyond corporate marketplace manipulation, Medicare, and insurance company rules, there are a host of other legislative forces to be reckoned with. As the health care giant grew, it lurched forward regurgitating increasingly onerous rules and regulations. Politically generated legislation like HIPPA (Health Information Portability and Accountability Act)—intended to protect medical confidentiality, electronic record requirements designed to promote communications, and the Affordable Care Act have each added cost and complexity without solving problems to anyone's satisfaction.

HIPPA's focus was protecting patient records and confidentiality, perceived to be threatened by an increasingly technological world. Nice idea, but on the way to dealing with a relatively straightforward problem, a law emerged that added draconian regulations and penalties, all of it obscured in a cloud of unreadable legalese. Along with a herd of lawyers newly specializing in HIPPA law, the educational seminar industry stepped up with programs to decipher the law and spell out how to maintain compliance.

There is a Murphy-like law at work in all of these interlocking overhauls of reason: blending legislative speed with complexity always breeds confusion instead of clarity. The Americans with Disabilities Act is another good example. The rules are convoluted, penalties severe, specialists interpreting the law are everywhere, and inevitably the Supreme Court was sucked in to tell us what the law *really* means.

Back in the late 1960s, we were only vaguely aware that expanding legislation would gradually seep into every aspect of health care delivery. For us, it was still about learning our profession. We assumed that whatever happened, good judgment and a little malpractice insurance would see us through.

Who would have guessed how radically training and care were to change, and in the process, turn health care into a mechanized corporate enterprise leaving patients in the dust? We were taught that practicing medicine is an art as well as a science, that one had certain sacred obligations to patients and each other. The idea that physicians would aggregate under a corporate banner, advertise, and see their practice as a business wasn't on anyone's radar.

But in spite of the idea the elegance of our craft has been pushed aside by an assembly-line mentality, insurance nightmares, malpractice paranoia, and penalties dripping from the consequences of incontinent legislation, who would argue we are not better off today with instantly available scanning technology, detailed laboratory work, cancer screening, and treatments only dreamed of in the 1960s?

To be sure, there is among many of my older colleagues nostalgia for the time one actually felt a patient's pulse, percussed (using fingers to tap) chest and abdomen to determine what lay beneath, and routinely did a detailed neurologic examination without thinking it exceptional. Today, a "complete" physical is done in a few minutes. Even a neurological "exam" is nothing more than flashing a light at the pupils and a quick tap of the knees to elicit a telling reflex jerk. It speaks to a shift toward speed at the expense of caution, pressure to move money-making units down the track, each larded with as many billable procedures as possible, supported by an unspoken trust in technology to catch any real problems.

During one of those quickie examinations a few years ago, I rather meanly made one knee jerk more than the other. The doctor didn't notice and went straight for his latex glove. Had I spoken of something even modestly suggestive of a possible nervous system disorder, I would have immediately been referred for a neurology consultation. No need to try to figure that one out in the time allowed—too easy to miss something that could come back to bite you.

We used to have an alerting mantra, a way to encourage us to look for exceptions in even the most straightforward situation: "When you hear hoof beats in the street, remember, every once in a while, a zebra goes by." Today, the mantra reads: "When you hear hoof beats in the street, remember, every once in a while, a lawyer rides by on a zebra."

But don't imagine we always relied on diagnostic acuity and never on testing. However, we were more cautious about ordering tests, starting with the fact the cost of testing usually fell to the patient. Tests were rarely done quickly or painlessly. All needles—injection, IV, spinal, the whole lot—were fat, hollow stainless-steel nails topped with large square hubs, menacing by any standard. Today, needles are thin-walled, making the lumen (tunnel) of the needle larger for easier flow. A 22-gauge needle (standard size for drawing blood) is the same diameter as its 1960 grandfather, but it is significantly less painful to get stuck with today's model. Why? Because the thin wall is super sharp, offers less resistance as it penetrates, and the blood flows faster through the wider tunnel. Put it another way: if you sharpened two identical 22-gauge nails, then hollowed out each, one with thick walls and one with thin walls, which one would be more painful? Happily, the transition from hand-sharpened nails to disposable needles and plastic syringes was complete by the mid-1960s.

A parallel improvement was the introduction of suction tubes with disposable needles for drawing blood. Before, we used large glass syringes to draw blood, then squirted it into various tubes, some empty and meant to clot, others containing chemicals to prevent clotting. There was a chance of damaging red cells by exerting too much pressure on the narrow-lumen needles, ruining the entire sample, wasting time, and subjecting the patient to repeated sticks.

Today, we enjoy the luxury of instant test results because everything is automated, and tests take less time (and skill) to set up and run. Contrast that with the time when precious few automated lab systems were in place. Even a simple blood count was done by hand. As a medical student or intern, one was expected to be able to go to the lab and do a basic blood count and urinalysis, start a culture, stain and examine a sputum sample to identify specific bacteria or fungi, then return to the floor and start targeted treatment.

Then there is the wince factor: many of the tests were a lot more grueling than they are today. Sigmoidoscopy (examination of the last third of the large intestine) was done with a long, fat, rigid metal tube; worse, no one thought of using sedation for this highly unpleasant, often painful, procedure until well into the 1970s. The same was true of a host of other tests and procedures: they were done without a hint of anesthesia.

Spinal taps were routine, and heaven help you if there was suspicion of a brain tumor. No CT scan for you; instead, a "Pneumoencephalogram" was ordered. The poor patient was strapped sitting up in a metal cage, head trapped in a sling. A spinal needle was pushed into his back, spinal fluid withdrawn and replaced with air that would bubble up through the spinal column into his head creating contrast that would sometimes show up on an x-ray. The entire contraption was then spun around to move the air into particular parts of the brain.

Today, the same fellow would spend a few painless minutes in a CT scanner that would instantly produce a series of crystal-clear images.

In our day, medical students, interns, and residents drew the blood, started the IVs, and didn't hesitate to "cut down" to a hidden vein in urgent situations. We quickly learned to do a "femoral stick" (get blood from deep in the groin) when other veins weren't functioning, spinal tap, or—in an emergency—perform a tracheotomy (opening the breathing tube in the neck).

Today, all of those jobs are handled by a fleet of phlebotomists, IV specialists, and surgeons. In fact, medical students are no longer even taught those skills, a real blow to nostalgia. But while there might be some cache in doing the work ourselves, having teams who do nothing else is certainly more efficient. EMTs do spectacular emergency work in stressful, often dangerous situations. "Hospitalists" have largely replaced outpatient physicians who used to admit their own patients and see to their care—even at night. Nurses no longer make beds or empty bed pans, freeing them to do the more technical work for which they are trained.

The list goes on. Efficiency has narrowed the scope of one's training and duties at every level of patient care. The danger, it seems to me, is taking it too far, mechanizing and dehumanizing health care delivery to the point that the patient's concerns, and even the basics of personal history, will be lost. Content is distilled into abbreviated checklists that either distort answers or miss basic information altogether.

When you check in to see your doctor, you have to sign a clutch of legal documents giving permission for treatment, deciding who can see your notes, describing HIPPA rules, and of course, granting insurance companies unfettered access to everything about you. Then there will be a page or so of check lists, over-condensed "yes" and "no" answers that will become the backbone of your medical history.

The patient's history is the single most important part of every evaluation. It is designed to flow evenly through the details of your problem, connecting everything together to focus the physical and laboratory work needed for diagnosis and treatment. It is a basic document one refers to and updates at every opportunity.

Or at least it should. But, sadly, the sped-up, quickie history protocol of today simply doesn't capture those data needed to properly evaluate each individual patient. It's all about odds: forget zebras, go for the obvious, and only if that doesn't work out (and the insurance company is willing) does one need to look deeper. Brutal efficiency.

In defense of spending more energy on CYA (cover your ass) releases and HIPPA forms, you might assert it is necessary because we live in litigious times, and fear of being sued is to blame, not the medical profession. *You didn't have to worry about lawsuits back when you were in training; you don't get it.*

Only partly true. You might be surprised to know that the threat of lawsuits was real then, too, and frequently just as manipulative as today, though on a different scale, and with a different approach. Physicians were held in higher esteem in the past, and patients didn't automatically see any perceived error as an opportunity to cash in. Lawyers didn't advertise the good news of medical misfortune, and when they did sue, there was a high probability of the case going to trial.

Today, the strategy has shifted to settlement as opposed to trial. Situations that don't remotely merit a lawsuit are presented in a menacing way, threatening to cost the physician time and income and the malpractice carrier with expensive allocation of resources. So, settle it and move on.

While suits were far less common fifty years ago, they were still a fact of life; so much so, that third year medical students—at least in my school—were required to attend at least one malpractice trial. I doubt that practice continues today.

The defendant in the case I witnessed was Chairman of the Department of Medicine at a large teaching hospital. He was a widely known expert on Rheumatic Fever (RF), a highly prevalent and often deadly disease, one we all kept on our radar at all times. He presided over a large group of residents, and his Rheumatic Fever clinic and inpatient service were always full.

The case was about a returning RF patient admitted for treatment just as she had been many times before. Physical exams were done, her past records reviewed, and a treatment program outlined, starting with IV penicillin, a drug she had taken intermittently for several years. Suddenly, and inexplicably, she had a massive allergic reaction and died.

The family skipped over the hospital and its residents, instead going after the chairman, even though he had never met the patient and was not directly involved in her care. Those responsibilities were shouldered by a group of attending physicians and their residents. But the chief of service presumably had the deepest pockets, so he was the target.

The chairman's lawyer tried to get him to settle the case, but he refused for all the obvious reasons, most especially the fact the patient had taken penicillin many times before without incident. How could an anomalous allergic reaction be anticipated? More to the point, how could such an atypical event be considered wrongful?

When it came time for summation, the Chairman's lawyer offered a bland but thoroughly factual explanation of the science involved, all of it supported by a group of experts who had testified there was no reasonable way the woman's reaction could have been anticipated. Watching from the gallery, it was clear the jury was barely listening.

But when the plaintiff's lawyer got up, he didn't even bother to deal with the science, he went straight for the jugular. He leaned into the jury box, stared at each juror, and when he had their attention, turned and pointed to the Chairman and said, "Malpractice! It's as clear as the nose on your face." Then he looked over to the gallery at the patient's teenage daughter. "And, ladies and gentlemen of the jury, because of *him*, her mom won't be there to pin the corsage onto her prom dress." He was almost in tears at the thought.

I didn't stay for the conclusion, but it took about an hour to convict the Chairman of malpractice. This is not an exaggeration of what happened. I can still see it; it made an enormous impression on me.

Medical students today are keenly aware of the potential for malpractice lawsuits, something many now see as inevitable. For us, even the threat of a suit was a crushing event—at best a terrible embarrassment; at worst, the humiliation of being dragged into court. Today, "suits" are more often probes, feints whose purpose is to see how likely an insurance company is to settle. For lawyers, it is more profitable to pile up a series of modest settlements than it is to take a chance on a prom dress trial. For insurance companies, it's the same calculation as readmissions and interrupted treatment: simply the cheaper route to resolution.

And for the physician? It is an unsettling experience, a costly embarrassment, and something to be explained on every application for hospital privileges or participation on insurance panels. It's the shadow that follows you even in the dark. The only solace is that because the likelihood of being sued has become so commonplace, it has lost some of its sting.

The best protection against lawsuits has not, however, changed that much. The rules are simple: document everything repeatedly in the clearest terms, make a habit of consulting and recording the advice of colleagues, and follow HIPPA rules to the letter. And those release forms? They don't mean a thing in the hands of a persistent lawyer. They only acquire meaning when the record shows you actually took the time to go over pivotal parts, most especially anything known about side effects and possible complications of even simple procedures. But even that isn't enough without specific quotes from the patient. That means statements like, "The patient said..." Or: "The patient asked about...and I said..." Only then is there a chance your interaction over the release forms will have some meaning.

There is another tripwire in our litigious world: Policies and Procedures. Today's physician knows to stick like glue to all policies and procedures related to the workplace. To prove malpractice, both negligence and harm must be demonstrated, both quite difficult to prove, especially when expert witnesses disagree. But a persistent lawyer will search for small and seemingly insignificant deviations from written policy or procedure, turning each into an act of raging incompetence, and by inference: malpractice.

A Boston lawyer speaking to a group of physicians a few years ago made the point by saying, "A good lawyer can make any signed document into toilet paper, and turn Mother Teresa into an ax murderer." That confirmed my definition of a lawyer:

Law-yer: noun; a distortionist skilled in finding imaginary causal pathways between mishap and money.

The ground has steadily shifted under the entire world of health care delivery, not simply in the way physicians practice medicine, but also in the deployment of a vast array of interconnected, often invisible technical, legal, and financial systems. Its complexity is way beyond comparisons between five-cent candy bars and CT machines, or hands-on chest tappers and today's tech-dependent practitioners.

Most of my narrative will focus on training when the art of medicine began to yield to innovation in science and technology. We were just starting to see organ transplants become a reality, and the possibility of curing certain cancers was moving from fantasy to impending reality. Once started, change gathered speed and complexity. There was no going back. One could compare it to the end of the Old West when cowboys and outlaws had to give way to railroads and barbed wire fences. There is certainly nostalgia for some parts of the old system, but no one would seriously lobby for the return of hijacking gold from stagecoaches or stealing livers from accident victims.

I have altered some of the stories enough to protect individual patients, hopefully preventing anyone recognizing or being embarrassed by what I reveal. There are a few spots when such disguises are not possible without losing the impact of the story; however, those few cases are about remarkable people who might actually be pleased to know someone remembers and wants to tell their story. In one case, I found the patient 45 years after the fact and got permission to tell her story. Everything I describe is real, truthful, happened as I said it did, and any cover is only to protect patients, colleagues, and teachers without distorting or exaggerating the truth.

A quick word about gender pronouns. Most of what I write about took place before there was awareness or sensitivity about gender pronouns. Male was the go-to convention because it was, quite frankly, a male dominated world, particularly in medicine where women were hugely underrepresented. The exceptions were pediatrics and, to a lesser extent, psychiatry. The majority of medical students and faculty were male. The most extreme case was my own medical school, a males-only institution until 1961, a year after my class started. We jokingly referred to ourselves as the last class with hair on its chest. I know: gag me, horrible male pigs, but it was the zeitgeist of the time. The decision to admit women was greeted with a howl of protest from alumni who saw it as a sign the end was near.

The prevailing assumption was that women could not be depended on to fully utilize their training because of the inevitable distractions of marriage, pregnancy, and childcare. Even menstruation was thought to be a recurring impediment to learning and practice. Better to focus precious resources on men.

The all-men idea was part of my life from the third grade on, all the way through medical school. As bizarre as it sounds, with only one lonely exception—a school employee's daughter allowed in the fifth grade—I never had a class year with a female student. And I was not alone, at least through the end of college. Granted, extending the absurdity through medical school was an anomaly even at that time.

When writing about my time in school and the military, male forms dominate because that literally was the way it unfolded. Women were part of my experience in internship and residency, and my pronouns follow the story. Where speaking in more general terms, using only one gender form seemed needlessly rigid, and "his/her" looks and feels like the sterile and awkward bow to correctness it is. So, I use the form that feels most appropriate, and where that doesn't work, I flipped a coin.

By the way, Father William, I've figured out how you can balance an eel on the end of your nose: freeze it first.

2

GETTING STARTED—BADLY

IT WAS THE EXCEPTIONAL MEDICAL student who did not have a clear fix on the path to medical school even before starting college. Many had parents or close relatives in the profession, while others were drawn by their love of science, the influence of a personal medical experience, or that threatened commodity: a wish to serve. Many saw it as a way to make a comfortable living. And, yes, quite a few (though they might not admit it) liked the idea of being looked up to, maybe even sport an "MD" license plate so everyone would know, including the police who were less likely to stop a car with an MD plate.

Professional income was then relatively high, members got mortgages based solely on their medical degree, and physicians treated other physicians and their immediate family members without charge. Whether by tradition, comfort, or scientific satisfaction, it was a great career choice pursued with clear-eyed determination.

For me, it was None of the Above.

My decision to become a physician was made on impulse when I was nine. After surviving a two-month stretch at a New Hampshire summer camp, I returned home expecting to spend August on the Jersey shore with my parents, fishing, swimming, and relaxing on the beach without being yelled at by irritable camp counselors.

But my parents decided it would be better if I finished off the summer with my grandmother on her horse farm in western Virginia while they spent August traveling, free of the annoying responsibility of keeping an eye on me. Camp was bad enough, but nothing compared to life with my humorless, puritanical, snobby, rule-bound grandmother.

Fortunately, she had little use for me, preferring to spend every day with friends playing golf or bridge at the nearby Homestead Hotel. That left me free to roam the farm and hang around with the "locals," as my grandmother termed anyone who didn't own a set of Patty Berg golf clubs.

As soon as Grandmother's Rolls cleared the driveway, I headed up the hollow to Granny Cleek's place at the end of the two-mile dirt road. She not only tolerated me, but quickly became my friend and teacher. We gardened, pulled weeds, made lye soap, killed and plucked chickens, hauled water from the well, made butter, and washed clothes. She told me stories about the old days before tractors, electricity, or even cars came to the hollow, and when her friend Edna showed up with her guitar, we sat on the porch and listened while she played old mountain songs and hymns. It was heaven.

One day, Granny asked me what I was going to do when I grew up. I didn't have a clue, but clearly an answer was needed, so I blurted out, "I'm going to be a doctor."

She seemed distressed with my answer, and I later found out why. Her daughter, Dorothy, had overcome enormous obstacles to become a nurse, a nearly impossible achievement for a poor country girl in the 1920s living four walking miles over the mountain from the school bus stop. Sadly, just after graduation she developed tuberculosis, and two years later died in the cabin at the end of the long dirt road.

During a later visit, Granny gave me her daughter's 1929 medical dictionary, saying if I intended to become a doctor, I would need that book.

It was a promise I simply could not break. That was it. No

legacy, no drive to help mankind, not a clue in this world what I was getting into, it was just a promise.

Shortly after arriving at Yale in the fall of 1956, I met with my faculty advisor, a junior, junior dean of something, to plot my academic course. He started by asking if I had any idea what my major would be. When I said I intended to be in the premed program, he held up his hand like traffic cop, sighed wearily, and said, "'Premed' is not a program. It just indicates you plan to go to medical school."

The deflation continued. He didn't give a fig about my motivation; rather, he was more concerned that I not fall into the science major trap. In his view, anyone focusing exclusively on science courses in anticipation of a medical career risked squandering the chance for a truly broad liberal education. Part of the reason for his apparent disdain for anything "premed" was certainly academic elitism, though there was another reason.

Until 1962, the standard medical school admissions test (now known as the "MCAT") was the Modified Moss Test, a four-part test yielding a single combined score. The subtests were "Verbal Ability," "Quantitative Ability," "Science Achievement," and "Understanding Modern Society." Thus, freighting your years with science courses could actually work against you. Put it the other way around: an English major could score well on three of the four parts and bury a weak science performance in the aggregate score.

So, the dean was right about there being no immediate handicap for a liberal arts major. But he took it too far, not realizing that the same medical school that might be bamboozled by the Moss Test *expected* you to have already studied math, statistics, and have more than a passing acquaintance with genetics and basic physiology.

In the 1970s, the MCAT shifted both content and scoring in order to highlight individual science scores, particularly in chemistry, physics, and biology. "Understanding Modern Society" was out, proficiency in science was in. English majors were still welcome to apply, but there had better be a lot of science sandwiched between *Candide* and *Hamlet*.

Then there was my little problem with mathematics. I hated math, never had a knack for it, and after I finished algebra and geometry in prep school, I never took another math class. Not trigonometry, not solid geometry, and certainly not calculus. The dean didn't seem to think I needed to trouble my curriculum with math, probably the single worst piece of advice dispensed that day. It came back to haunt me in a big way in medical school.

Freshman year went by easily, the idea of medical school still on the distant horizon. But in the second year, my plan started to unravel. I found myself defending my anemic science program in conversation with other premed classmates, almost without exception science majors.

I tried to repair some of the damage by taking physics and chemistry at the same time. The (predictable) result was my first major academic disruption, especially in chemistry, taught by the oldest professor in the department, Dr. Brinkley. It was basic stuff, should have been easy enough, especially compared to organic chemistry looming on the horizon in junior year. But physics also demanded a lot of attention, and I quickly started to sink in Dr. Brinkley's class, bumping along with a dismal C average. After one particularly wretched test performance, Dr. Brinkley summoned me to his office to dispense some rather blunt advice.

"I taught your father when he was here, and he was no better than you are. I even caught him trying to cut my class one day. He sent someone to sit in his seat and thought I wouldn't notice. It doesn't look like the apple has fallen far from the tree." He finished me off by saying, "I understand you want to go to medical school. My advice is to forget about it. You'll never make it."

I checked with my father who confirmed his own struggle with chemistry, even the part about cutting Brinkley's class, a serious offense in 1932.

At first, I was devastated. I went back and forth between humiliation and anger. Fortunately, the anger part won. I doubled down on chemistry, managing to escape with a gentlemanly B minus, but not without a lot of soul searching about the entire medical school idea. Did I have the right stuff to make it? Was a promise made at the age of nine a real motivator or just a romantic fantasy? And what did I really know about a medical career, anyway?

I could no longer sell myself on the idea of sticking to my promise to Granny. It was fine for a kid plucking chickens and ducking his evil grandmother, but this was about choosing one's life work. It demanded a sober decision based on a match of options and ability, and at that point, the ability part seemed rather shaky. In fact, no career choice of any sort really stood out.

My personal experiences with doctors had not been particularly positive, especially the two surgeries I had as a kid, both with the world's most awful anesthetic: ether. The first was a tonsillectomy at age four, something almost all kids underwent as a matter of course before starting school. Kids often went to the hospital in groups just to make it all more fun. I remember being held down and smothered with ether, waking up, smelling it, and instantly puking.

The second time was when my appendix exploded at a Christmas party at my rotten grandmother's house. Again, I was held down, a metal mask clamped to my face while ether was dripped into the contraption. Again, more puking.

My point is, while I was repulsed by the idea of life with a slide rule in my father's engineering business, I wasn't really drawn toward medicine, certainly not with the zeal of my premed classmates. Still, there was a clear fascination with the idea of being part of a constantly evolving profession, as opposed to seemingly static occupations like law, economics, and teaching. Except for a distant aunt on my mother's side who started a medical school in India,[1] I had no family ties to anything even vaguely medical.

---

1. Ida A. Scudder (1870–1960) was born in India, the granddaughter of the first American missionary to India. She graduated from Cornell Medical School in 1899, part of the first Cornell class to accept women. She returned to Vellore, India, where she dared to provide

interesting fact

I hadn't even had a serious conversation with a physician about the feasibility of my plan.

My parents were no help, either. Mother liked the idea largely because it would keep me out of Father's business. But that idea was a goner anyway because of my nonexistent math skills. For his part, Father was phobic about anything medical, worried incessantly about the latest disease, and mention of words like "blood," "pus," or "gangrene" would infuriate him. No help there.

Clearly, I had to figure this out on my own—and in a hurry. Committing to medicine meant sharpening my focus, working a lot harder to get the grades and learn what I would need—all before it was literally too late, and I would have to turn to something else, like psychology or even law school.

Go to the source, I reasoned. Yale had a medical school affiliated with Grace New Haven Hospital, so I made an appointment hoping to get some objective advice. It took a few false starts before I was able to convince the appointment censors I wasn't another undergraduate trying to maneuver an early application interview. I ended up with a junior, junior dean who listened deadpan to my feeble story. He called the whole thing thin soup, especially the part about exiling mathematics from my academic plan.

But what really seemed to get his attention was my complete lack of understanding of what the profession was all about. So, he had a suggestion: before trying to bring the torment of math back into the picture, I should join a group called the Yale Aids and get exposed to hospital life at Grace New Haven, meet some medical students, and see if I wanted to swap sentimental commitment for the real thing.

It was a good piece of advice, though at first it didn't seem like more than volunteering to be a medical janitor running errands

---

medical care for women, and in 1918, she and her surgeon niece, Ida B. Scudder, started a teaching hospital for women. Today, it is one of the country's great clinical centers, known for research and treatment of tropical diseases.

and cleaning up messes the regular aids wouldn't touch. There was also the problem of time. I needed all the time I could muster to keep my head focused on grades, and that left precious little time for bedpans, even if my future was somehow on the line.

But I stuck at it, mostly on weekends, sometimes late nights when I didn't have early morning class. Slowly, the enormous hospital started to make sense, along with a rudimentary understanding of the hierarchy and protocols one had to master in order to blend in with something approaching comfort.

Unfortunately, the medical students were too busy and too far up the ladder to bother with a lowly aide in a silly blue coat, and I was totally invisible to interns, residents, and the teaching faculty. This was learning by observation, but I saw a lot.

The best show in town was "Making Rounds," a full-on production held twice a day, led by an "Attending" (faculty member) to both teach and review each case on the Attending's ward. The train left the nurses' station with the most senior resident leading the way, followed by the Attending, then the head nurse, all three just in front of the large rolling chart rack pushed along by a medical student, followed by residents arranged by year, then the interns, and finally by a mix of nurses and medical students.

It was a solemn procession focused primarily on the interaction between the Attending and his residents. At each bedside, one of the residents would present a brief summary of the case, then the grilling began. Most of the questions were fired at residents and interns, but sometimes he would ambush a medical student. You never knew when your number would be called, and you had better be ready with the right answer.

Some Attendings were fatherly and only seemed interested in teaching. Others were outright bored and only came to life when something curious or unusual came up. But quite a few were downright caustic, seeming to delight in tripping up the unprepared.

My position was that of the circus worker following the elephants into the center ring, just close enough to pick up the droppings, but far enough back not to be seen as part of the act, or worse: get dumped on.

Several months passed without any close encounters with death. There were some anxious moments, to be sure, all glimpsed from the background, but no one had died while I was on duty. That changed one evening at the height of visiting time. A family member reported to the nurse that her father seemed not to be responding and asked if she would check. The patient was in a double room, against the far wall, a curtain separating the two patients.

The nurse checked the man's pulse, then almost casually turned to the two visitors and asked if they would kindly step out in the hall. "He's dead," she mouthed silently to me, then asked if I would please call the intern and the hospital chaplain. The intern confirmed the situation, the family was taken to the quiet end of the hall where the chaplain broke the news, and together they left for the chapel.

I had never before seen a dead person. Even when my grandfather died when I was a kid, they had him boxed up immediately, and I was spared the experience, left to wonder what he might look like in death.

The nurses were very busy at that particular time, no medical students were around, and the intern quickly disappeared. That left me with the nurse.

"We have a problem," she whispered. "We need to get him down to the morgue as quickly as possible, but we don't want to parade him in front of visitors and the other patients." She said that seeing someone wheeled by with a sheet over his head was unsettling, and we had to come up with another plan. Waiting two hours for visitors to leave was a not an option. I suggested we leave the IV in his arm, then whisk him quickly down the hall with his face sort of but not quite covered. Another patient going for an x-ray, who would notice?

She nixed the IV but bought the casual push down the hallway. The man was quite heavy, and it took a while to get him onto the gurney, more a rolling stretcher than the high-tech devices we know today. With the sheet in place, we set sail, managing the turn into the hallway fairly easily, but at that moment, the nurse was called away, leaving me to carry on.

By protocol, a deceased person was transported to the morgue using the freight elevator at the end of the unit, a fair distance from our starting point. The nurse had been at the head of the gurney, and thinking it might be a waste of time to switch places, I started to push my load down the hall. It was a mistake.

Because most of the weight was at the other end of the gurney, it wouldn't track straight ahead, and started to sway from one side to the other. I quickly switched ends, but I still couldn't get the wheels to cooperate. As I fishtailed down the hallway, people had to dodge into doorways to get out of the way. I'm sure they felt badly for the poor patient being rocked back and forth. Regrettably, the swerving motion was pulling the sheet out of place, exposing his face, eyes closed and mouth hanging open like a torn pocket.

I finally cleared the room area, got to the elevator, and pushed the down button. Unfortunately, every time it stopped, it was full of maintenance people, clerks, and laundry carts, so I had to wait for another round trip. I was sweating, my heart was pounding, and I was terrified someone would see I was pushing a corpse, call security, and get me thrown out along with any hope of a medical career. I finally got an empty elevator, but while trying to get the gurney on board in a more-or-less straight line, the impatient doors closed on the gurney pulling the sheet almost completely off the patient. I managed to get in, hit the button for the basement, and start to get the sheet back together when the elevator stopped, and a nurses' aide stepped on.

"What are you doing with a patient on the freight elevator?!" she demanded. Then she looked a little closer at the man's face. "Oh, my God! He's dead. What the hell are you doing?!"

"I'm going to the morgue. Maybe you could help." Weak, but the best I could do at the moment. She got off at the next floor without saying a word, just looked back at me with a mix of contempt and horror. Finally, I got to the basement, gave a mighty shove, and cleared the elevator without getting bitten by the doors.

I was alone in the hallway, so I took a minute to catch my breath. Almost there, I thought. I just wanted to adjust the sheet, get down the hall, deliver the body, and get out of there.

But as I pulled the sheet up again to cover his face, I saw his eyes had opened about halfway, and he was staring at me. Another awful moment. Was he still alive? Do I call someone? The best course of action seemed to be to go straightaway to the morgue and let them deal with it.

Because I had never been to the morgue before, I had no idea if I was going in the right direction. In my distraction, I made a wrong turn, came to a large steel door, switched ends, and backed through, paying more attention to the door than what was behind me. I did think it was mighty cold in there, but that's the nature of morgues, I reasoned. I cleared the door, it snapped shut, and I turned around expecting to see a morgue attendant. Not so. I found myself alone in a room opening onto a loading dock. It was cold, late at night, no one was around, and the door was locked. I couldn't very well leave the body on the loading dock while I went for help. But standing there in the cold waiting for Godot didn't seem like a really great option, either.

After a few very bad few minutes, I noticed a metal box on the wall and, inside, a telephone—and it was working! I asked to be connected with the morgue, told the attendant I had a body on the loading dock and would he please hurry up.

The attendant was full of questions, but feeling like all three Stooges combined, I was in no mood to talk. I handed him the chart and turned to leave.

"Hey! Where do you think you're going?"

"Home."

"Not until you help me move this body and return the gurney."

I made it back without running over anyone and left the gurney by the nurses' station.

"What took you so long?" asked the nurse who had sent me off on the hellish journey.

"We went out for a drink."

Fortunately, she only rolled her eyes, and I was off the hook.

Walking home, I couldn't shake the image of the loading dock and the dead man staring at me. It felt like he was saying, "Are you kidding me? *You?* A *doctor?* You can't even find the morgue." Quit? Go on? Back and forth it went. Then I started to think about all the characters in the huge play I had been watching at Grace New Haven. They seemed so determined not to just play their parts, but to do so flawlessly, often under grueling conditions. And in the end, they made a difference. Clearly, that was behind it all.

Granny's daughter, Dorothy, had the same drive. She walked over a mountain—no matter the weather—to complete high school. She left home to go to nursing school, then moved to Chicago to start her career. She didn't limp away just because of some embarrassing misstep. Maybe all my obsessing really came down to a fairly simple question: are you willing to push yourself into an uncomfortable place, take a chance you might fail, in order to do something that might actually have some meaning? The answer was still, "Maybe," but a month later the matter was settled; again, it had to do with taking a body to the morgue.

Normally, the Emergency Department was an area assigned to more senior Aides. It was fast paced, highly organized, and everybody knew exactly how to move with the flow. It was not for the uninitiated. But one Sunday night, I was told to go to the ER because the scheduled Aide couldn't make it. Besides, it was a slow night and a good time to learn some of the fundamentals.

I was given a fast tour by a nurse, told what my duties would be, encouraged to watch, and above all: stay out of the way. At that point a call came in from the police saying there had been an accident on the Merritt Parkway, two men involved, one seriously injured, and the other deceased. The on-call surgeon was notified, and soon several residents and interns arrived. A nurse and two orderlies were ready at the door.

Two ambulances arrived, the one with the injured man well ahead of the other. As the stretcher was rolled through the door, the intern and nurse started to rip the man's clothing away from an enormous chest wound. The stretcher continued into the surgical bay, and I was told to wait for the second ambulance. That stretcher was rolled in almost casually, the body covered by a blood-soaked sheet. A nurse looked under the sheet and directed the ambulance drivers to a vacant treatment bay. I was told to help the orderly move the body onto a hospital gurney so the ambulance people could have their stretcher back. OK, brace yourself, I remember thinking. You can do this. But I almost didn't, because when the sheet was pulled back, I saw that although the man was on his back, his head was at more than a ninety-degree angle to the body. In fact, he was nearly decapitated, his head barely left attached to the body. It was a jolt I can still remember.

We moved the body into a body bag, zipped it up, and I was told to deliver it to the morgue. When I got back from the morgue, I was dispatched to the blood bank for several pints of blood. The tone was businesslike but urgent, and I moved as fast as I could, all the while thinking I might be holding the man's life in my hands.

The drama went on for an hour, a group of physicians crowded around the table tying off bleeders, trying to maintain breathing and blood pressure. Finally, the chief surgeon said over his shoulder to no one in particular, "Better call the priest."

The holy man showed up in less than fifteen minutes, kissed and donned a shawl, got out a bottle of oil, then leaned into the group near the man's head, and said, "Mario, are you sorry for your sins?"

Mario had been drifting in and out of semi-consciousness, but in that moment, he seemed to hear, and said, "I'll say anything!" The priest reached in, anointed his forehead, said something in Latin, and left. A few minutes later Mario was gone.

Everyone stopped. There was a long moment of silence, no one moved at all. Then the surgeon peeled off his gloves, dropped them on the man's chest, and muttered, "You can't win them all."

He pulled off his bloody gown, dumped it in a hamper, and left. The others followed suit.

That left the head nurse, the orderly, and me with Mario.

"Pull out all the needles, cannulas, and tubes. Put all the instruments in the tray, put him in a bag, and take him to the morgue," the nurse said as she, too, shed her soiled gown and left.

The orderly was perfectly aware of my distress and dealt with it by telling me to get busy with the tubes while he prepared the bag. Needles and cannulas that only minutes before had been Mario's connection to life were suddenly nothing more than contaminated instruments headed for the autoclave room to be cleaned, sterilized, wrapped, and put back on the shelf. Maybe the next patient will be luckier than Mario.

It would overwork the memory to say it was transforming, or that any of the other times I was exposed to life and death drama in that hospital had set me on a determined path toward medicine. But collectively, the experiences did convince me this was a world I could handle, one that answered questions I hadn't yet thought about, and I should definitely make a real effort to see if I could make it happen.

By that time, I was halfway through college, my grades were holding up, and I only had the Moss test and one more major course to get past: a bear called Organic Chemistry. With a decent grade, I at least had a shot; without it—time to rethink my options. The same is true today: Organic Chemistry is the pivot, the most important course for any premed student.

The course had a well-deserved reputation as both tough and time consuming. With mounting pressure from my somewhat neglected English major, upcoming junior year was shaping up as an all-work and no-play grind. I quit the Yale Aids to gain a little time, but what I really needed was an edge, something that would get me through it, and still have a social life.

I am going to take a detour in the narrative at this point to tell a story about an event in that social life, one that at first just seemed to be a cosmic anomaly unrelated to my putative medical career, but in a bizarre way, no matter how unlikely, it did have a slight but palpable effect on my training. This is Part One of the Tale of John Jesus.

It all started with a wildly popular North Carolina band, The Hot Nuts, a rock and roll band heavy on brass and dirty lyrics. They were so popular on the college fraternity circle, it was nearly impossible to get in to hear them without being a "brother." My good friend Stephen, at the University of Virginia (UVA), kept tabs on the group, and when they came to Charlottesville for a two-night stint, he managed to get us into one of the parties. I drove to Charlottesville, and with drunken exuberance, stomped, and sang away the night to the group's hit songs: "Hot nuts! Hot nuts! Get 'em from the Peanut Man," and "He's Got the Whole World by the Balls."

The next morning, we went to the University Diner to sooth our hangovers. I was rehydrating in anticipation of the seven-hour trip back to New Haven, thinking about the paper I still had to write that night. Suddenly, an emaciated white man waving a Bible loomed in the doorway yelling about the wages of sin and the need for immediate repentance! He moved quickly from table to table shaking the Bible in people's faces, but not getting any takers. But when he got our table, Stephen said if he would please stop yelling and sit down, we would be glad to buy him some food and hear his story.

He did sit, lowered his voice, and introduced himself as John Jesus, Preacher of the Gospel, Servant of the Lord, and no thanks, he didn't need food because, "The Lord fills my stomach with heavenly food." He opened his Bible and started to preach. Every single word in the entire book was individually underlined in red, its pages so thumb-worn one could hardly read the first word of each line. It didn't really matter, though, because John had it all memorized. Stephen managed to slow him down enough to learn that following divine direction, he was on an East Coast mission to save souls. Charlottesville was just one stop on his peregrination.

When I left, Stephen and John were still talking. As it turned out, that conversation took Stephen to the edge of expulsion from UVA. He was a philosophy major, and by chance, Archibald MacLeish, philosopher and theologian, was going to speak before a large group of students and faculty the next day. Would John be interested in attending? It might be interesting for him to hear the talk. John accepted, showed up, and sat in the back, promising Stephen he would listen in silence—maybe a question or two later.

They had a deal, though in reflection, "seemed" to have a deal would have been more accurate. Unfortunately, MacLeish began his talk on the fusion of theology and philosophy by saying that there was no absolute proof of the existence of God. Wham! John was on his feet, Bible held aloft, yelling that there certainly was proof of the existence of God! It took several campus cops to get John out. Stephen skulked back to his apartment terrified he would be found out, interrogated, and dismissed from school. Fortunately, it didn't happen, and the John Jesus chapter was closed. Or so we thought.

Back to Yale and the burning question of how to deal with the rising menace of Organic Chemistry. There was no concealing my mediocre performance in Brinkley's course, doubling the grade stakes in Organic. It somehow had to look like I had undergone some sort of chemistry epiphany, cured of my inorganic sins. The answer was to take Organic in summer school somewhere else. If I aced it, then transfer the grade and go back to Chaucer. If not, then don't say a word about summer school, take it again, and hope for a good grade without having to kill myself.

Rutgers University offered a summer course in its Newark, New Jersey, branch, conveniently close to home. I was optimistic about my plan until the professor walked into our first class. He wore a starched white lab coat and a look of seriousness that said the next eight weeks were not going to be anything like a walk in the park.

After silently scanning the group of perhaps thirty students, he said in a dead-flat tone: "My name is *Panson*, spelled backwards, that's *No-Snap*. And that's the way it's going to be."[2]

I wondered what it was about chemistry that sucked the optimism and humor out of people. Or was he somehow related to Dr. Brinkley? Either way, the prospect of repeating the course in junior year suddenly looked like a disturbing probability. I dug in, did reasonably well for the first half, but then Dr. Panson accelerated the pace, and I finished with a middling grade. Good enough for government work, but well short of the number I needed to fatten my academic record.

Back for junior year, I silently repeated Organic, got the grade I needed, and started to think Medical School might still be possible. I also signed up to audit Advanced Organic Chemistry in senior year, a rather transparent move to put a cherry on top of my melting sundae. I attended exactly one class, not out of indifference, but as a reaction to being told some of the research papers were in German. Hope no one minds. Attended or not, the audit still showed up on my transcript. Good enough. Another baited hook in the water.

By the fall of senior year, I was well acquainted with my fellow premeds, all of whom seemed to know everything there was to know about every medical school, to the point of being able to list them from the most competitive down to the least. I applied to eight schools, focusing on the ones with no mathematics requirement. Six invited me to an interview, a real morale booster until I realized that almost everyone was getting the same treatment. You had to be a real dud not to get at least one interview.

Among the premeds, the interview loomed as both promising and frightening. It was your chance to shine, stand out from

---

2.   Gilbert S. Panson (1920–2013). Graduated magna cum laude from Brown University, received his Master's and PhD in chemistry from Columbia University. He worked on the Manhattan Project, then became Professor of Chemistry and Dean and Chairman of the Department of Chemistry at Rutgers University (1946–1985).

the rest, but it was also a nowhere-to-hide chance to fall flat on your face. There were wild stories about devious, even sadistic, tactics used to throw an interviewee off his stride. One was said to ask the victim to open a window that had been wedged shut, a test of one's reaction under sudden stress. Another was to conduct the interview in a very hot or freezing cold room. Another was said to begin in absolute silence, the interviewer simply staring at you to see how you wriggled out of that one. We were cautioned to arrive early, check out exactly where to go to avoid yet another trick: odd appointment times coupled with vague directions; again, a test of one's ability to anticipate and deal with ambiguity.

My first interview was a nightmare. It started with a brief tour of the school by a bored medical student who displayed absolutely no interest in conversation, or even a sliver of advice about the interview. He dropped me off in a small, windowless hallway where I stood (there was no chair) and waited. Finally, one of the junior, junior deans arrived, introduced himself, invited me into an office, pointed to a chair, and started asking questions about where I was from, why I had chosen to apply to his school—all of it brusque—but nothing bone crushing.

Just as I was getting comfortable, he said he was going to give me a job. "Oh, shit! Here we go," I thought. The "job" was to describe how I would go about building an electron microscope. I mumbled something about needing a stream of electrons, tried to stretch it out, but it went nowhere. The interview lasted all of fifteen minutes, a disaster from the start. I had a long train ride back to New Haven, plenty of time to again wonder if this entire undertaking might not be a colossal mistake.

I don't recall much about the next four interviews, but I do recall feeling increasingly like someone going over Niagara Falls in a laundry basket. By the time I got to the sixth and final interview, I already had a rejection letter from Doctor Electron Microscope. I knew from the start it was a no-go, no surprise there, but I was taken aback by how quickly I was scratched. Even worse, acceptance letters were reaching others, and several were trying to pick between competing schools.

One to go. I didn't even bother to read up on electron microscopes. Screw it. Two careers down the drain: medicine and chemistry. The way things were going, I soon wouldn't even be able to add "English Teacher" to the list of possible careers.

The process was the same: a medical student tour, then the wait, but this time I was in a waiting room with other hopefuls, one from my class at Yale. The interviewer was actually pleasant, and after some small talk, he went straight to the heart of the matter: my major. But instead of sneering, he said he admired premed students who could balance liberal arts and science at the same time.

Then he said he had a test for me, a printed page with twenty words numbered down the left side. "It's a vocabulary test. I think every physician should be able to use language as well as manipulate numbers." I was to write a definition of each word, keep it simple, and don't take long.

I don't do electron microscopes or waterfalls, but I do have a reasonably good vocabulary, and I correctly defined all twenty words. He told me I was the first one to do it, and with that, the interview was over. A month later I received an acceptance letter from Jefferson Medical College. It seemed impossible, but it happened.

The letter was brief, I was accepted—congratulations—and if I wanted to attend please return the enclosed agreement promptly. Tuition was $500 a year, $750 for the first year to cover the cost of a cadaver. See you on September 12, 1960, more information to follow.

I hardly noticed the rest of senior year, though inattention to my English major was stirring some concern, and I was advised to add another literature course already well under way. Catching up was a problem, but I squeaked through, graduated, all the while wondering if I might become a victim of the old adage about getting what you wished for: you might regret it.

3

MEDICAL SCHOOL
PANSON'S AND BRINKLEY'S REVENGE

ABOUT A MONTH BEFORE CLASSES were to begin, I found a small apartment over an antique store just six blocks from the core of the medical school, just two blocks from the Daniel Baugh anatomy building where all classes were taught for the first five months of freshman year. Its isolation from the main campus made it feel like I had been accepted by a building, not a medical school, certainly not the grand fantasy I had back in college. Instead of walking around an Old Philadelphia campus luxuriant in ivy and tradition, I was to be confined to a nondescript three-story building, closeted with 176 classmates, 44 dead bodies, a phalanx of irritable teachers, all of it enveloped in the suffocating stench of formaldehyde.

I bought a microscope, required texts, several lab coats, and a dissection kit. The Zeiss microscope was an amazing instrument—well beyond any microscope I had ever used before. It cost the equivalent of two year's tuition. Using one of its specialized lenses and a drop of oil on top of a glass slide, one could peer into a single cell. Dissection and using the microscope became the two learning experiences I most looked forward to during the endless grind of that first year.

I set up my apartment and wondered what in the world to do next. The anatomy building was off limits until the first day of class, frustrating my plan to get acquainted with the layout ahead of the start of classes.

Happily, I ran into a number of other first year students and quickly realized that it would be smart to join a medical fraternity, not simply for social reasons, but as a place to take all of one's meals, meet others—including upper classmen—and generally begin to get some idea of what was coming, and how to deal with it.

Upper classmen seemed to delight in telling menacing tales of what lay ahead. Their first piece of advice: buy some oil of wintergreen, splash it on like after shave lotion to fight off the nauseating stench of body decomposition and formaldehyde. We were warned about the icy impatience of the anatomy teachers, killer exams, and embarrassing call-out questions thrown at random during lectures.

One helpful fellow summed it up by saying, "You go to class in the dark, you go home in the dark, and when you eat, please sit in the freshman corner of the dining room." Formaldehyde again.

But the most chilling of all facts was literally about seats; specifically, the number in the pathology lab in the second year. There were 152 seats in the pathology lab. That meant the bottom 24 of our class would be dropped at the end of the year even if they were passing everything. Slow starters not invited. As a slight consolation, a few would be invited to try again the following year, but the rest were simply canned.

We were told in a typically terse letter that class would begin Monday, September 12. Dress code: slacks, necktie, and white lab coat. Normally, class began at 7:30 a.m., but on the first day we were to report to the morgue in the basement (where else?) to pick up a box of bones and a skull. Doors to the morgue would open promptly at 6:30 a.m., first lecture to begin at 9:00 a.m. sharp. Bring your dissection kit. Nothing about good luck or have fun opening old stomachs.

Because everything seemed to run with such precision, I decided it would be prudent to be at the morgue ahead of time. "6:15 a.m. ought to do it," I thought. But when I walked through the front door, I was stunned to see there was already a line not only disappearing down the basement stairs but extending all the way to the back of the building, ending somewhere around the far corner. I finally got to the end, one of the last dozen or so to arrive. Images of the pathology lab seats flashed through my mind.

As if that wasn't strange enough, the place was deadly silent. A few who knew each other talked quietly, but most of the rest had their nose in the *Grant's Anatomy*, studying. *Studying?* Studying what? Had I missed something? Was there an assignment written in invisible ink in that letter about textbooks and microscopes?

I introduced myself to the two fellows next to me, but the conversation went nowhere. Awkwardly, I push on and asked where they had gone to college. One mumbled a name I missed entirely, the other said, "Thiel." I had never heard of Thiel College (a liberal arts Lutheran school in Greenville, Pennsylvania, established in 1866), and not wanting to look more foolish than I already was, I said, "Oh," implying I knew it well. The conversation was in free fall at that point, and the best I could do was ask what his major had been. He looked at me as if I was the perfect fool, and said, "Chemistry, really, but I did take comparative anatomy, physiology, and some histology." This time, the "Oh" was one of simple defeat. He went back to his book, and I continued to think I might just be living out the single biggest mistake of my life.

We later became friends, even to the point of joking about my clumsy start. He went on to a distinguished career in the Army Medical Corps, achieved the rank of General, but died in a training accident when his parachute failed to open.

At the time, I didn't quite know why my questions seemed so hopelessly naïve, but I later found out that many of my classmates were products of "premed colleges," institutions geared to both getting their students into medical school, as well as preparing them for the pending scientific onslaught. Some of the schools were considered feeder schools for specific medical schools. No matter; clearly, Yale wasn't in the medical school game.

For those clever enough to have followed the feeder path, most of freshman year was a review of what they had already learned. They were prepared all the way down to the new vocabulary we had to absorb, between 800 and 1,000 technical words in freshman year alone, not counting the names of specific anatomic structures. In *Grant's Anatomy*, there were 4,990, and in *Gray's Anatomy*, almost 10,000. To come up with the numbers, I counted what would have been new words on ten random index pages of the main first year texts, and did a little math even I can handle.

They also knew the teaching system of individual schools. Penn Medical was said to be gentlemanly and less confrontational than others, plus it had plenty of seats in its teaching labs. Harvard had already given up on testing, and was said to treat its students like future professors. Unfortunately, Jefferson was known for its blunt, unforgiving style, quirky professors, and constant testing.

Today, there is no line to the morgue. In fact, there is no morgue, not even anatomy class! Only students who specifically feel the need for anatomy take the course—as an elective. Why clutter your time with something you don't need? The anatomy of a specific organ or system can be mastered from books and demonstrations, dissection only as a last resort.

As we slowly made our way toward the basement steps, I got another realty jolt, this one a line of white poster boards taped to the front hall wall, the name of each student listed in alphabetical order indexed to a seemingly endless series of boxes extending across the boards. Atop each column, headings like, "Anat. Test #1," and "Hist. Test #2."

I was completely taken back by the idea everyone would see every grade. Passing grade was 75, and failing grades were written in red, a mark you could see ten feet away. The 75–79 range was in a nasty purple just to make the point it was not considered a worthy grade. Everything else was in black, to make the point this was where one was expected to be.

The system was alarming yet highly motivating, the scarlet numbers and the image of the missing 24 seats in the pathology lab a constant reminder one could not slack off for a second.

Another twist in the testing system quickly revealed itself: there was no gap between classes and major tests. Tests were generally given on Saturday, and one had a full day of classes the day before. And to be sure, there would be material on the test from Friday's lectures.

"Studying for finals" was suddenly a discarded relic, a radical departure from prep school and college based on the concept that as physicians in training we were expected to be in a constant state of review, ready at any minute to take a major exam. After all, that's what practice would be like: making instant decisions based on a constantly maintained fund of knowledge.

I cursed that Yale sub-dean who dismissed "premed" as an empty vessel, a distraction from the chance to get a real education. A lot of damn good it did to be able to read Chaucer in Old English when I was expected to stand up and describe some minute aspect of kidney function right out of the gate. The guy from Thiel could do it, but for me it was like being asked about the freaking electron microscope all over again.

In today's world, grades aren't considered important at all, and no instructor would dream of badgering a student in front of an entire class. In fact, the shoe is on the other foot: students evaluate teachers at the end of each course. There are tests, to be sure, but only to give a private, individual read on how one is progressing. And there are plenty of seats in the pathology lab. They probably have feather cushions, too.

One professor told me that today's students come in knowing exactly what their specialty will be. They disdain anything else, attend lectures when they feel like it, and have no difficulty with tests.

"They're smart, great at memorization, quickly master details, already have computer skills, and have made exam-cram a fine skill. They have zero interpersonal skills, and little interest in pathology or people. Their focus is entirely on procedures. We had to cut back on the number of lectures because of lack of attendance."

Interestingly, no two medical schools seem to have the same curriculum. They're all trying to figure out what works, what will engage students to learn basics like interviewing skills, how to take a history without a computer, and listen without constantly monitoring their cell phones.

One school tried to elevate empathy into students' awareness by offering a humanities class. One of the lectures was about Primo Levi, Jewish-Italian chemist, diabetes researcher, writer, and resistance fighter arrested in 1943 by Mussolini's secret police, sent to Auschwitz, then to Birkenau, from there to Russia after liberation, eventually making it back to Italy on foot. He told the story in his book *Survival in Auschwitz*.

"It failed completely. The ones who showed up didn't look up from their cell phones." The humanities course was dropped. The dean's assessment of medical education today: "We've lost it."

In defense of the newer, kinder system, another dean told me that being accepted meant the student is already assumed to be able and motivated to do the work, no sorting out necessary. Constant testing is seen as a distraction and a poor measure of learning compared with one's level of participation, "informed interaction," and self-assessment. A student sensing the need for help in a particular area has but to turn to colleagues or a friendly teacher. Besides, there are national tests to take one's measure. True: at the end of second year, medical students across the country take the National Board Examination, Part I, covering all aspects of basic medical science. Part II is given before graduation to review basic medical material and test medical skills. Part III at the end of the first postgraduate training year sums it all up, giving the green light to states to issue a medical license. There is a common misperception that licensing comes with graduation, but since 1915, successfully completing all three National Boards has been required first.

But the shift to anxiety-free instruction was way beyond my horizon that September morning in 1960. We were still in the grip of old school terror teaching, like relying on a hurricane to prune your fruit trees.

The line eventually reached the cellar stairs then fell into the emptiness below. Light pouring through first floor windows was replaced by overhead bulbs hanging in white metal funnels. The trip down was endless, like walking down the stairs into a London subway during a power outage. At the bottom, a yellow line and a sign in front of the open door to the morgue commanded, "Stay behind the line until you are called."

When it was my turn, I stepped into the gloom up to a counter illuminated by a single overhead light (lights generate heat, and in a giant icebox, heat is the enemy). Behind the counter stood a man wearing a wrap-around butcher's apron, a wool hat (it was very cold in there), and a scowl. He recorded my name, pushed the bone box and skull across the counter, and delivered a quick lecture on bone care punctuated with threats to my wellbeing if a pencil mark or the tiniest bit of damage should be found when I turned in the bones at the end of the year.

I was so preoccupied with the moment I didn't really take in the room itself beyond the fact it was huge, cold, dark, and reeked of death. I had the fleeting impression of amorphous shapes on steel tables tailing off into the gloom. We had been told by upper classmen to look into the freezer chest beyond the counter to see the body of a child dressed in a suit and tiny bow tie, alleged to be the mortician's private trophy and ghoulish reminder that we were transitioning into a world of new rules and realities.

I saw the open freezer, and maybe something in it, but in the excited buzz later about who saw what, I could contribute nothing. To this day, I don't know if the story was true, but as Theater of the Dead, it has us all in its grip.

Being at the end of the line meant I was also among the last to find a seat in the "pit," an enormous, steep-sided bullring where all lectures were given. I was near the top, two stories above the floor; at the bottom, a chalkboard on wheels and a lectern—nothing else. At exactly 9:00 a.m. a door opened and the matador, Dr. Burns, walked in, looked around briefly, and announced he would lecture until noon, break one hour for lunch, then we were to go to the anatomy lab to begin dissection.

Without breaking stride, he jumped straightaway into his talk saying we would begin work on the skin on the back just below the shoulder, six inches left of the spine. "That will reveal what muscle?" he demanded in a loud voice as he ran his finger down the list of names.

"Holy shit," I thought. "Now I see what all the studying was about. How had I missed it? More to the point, what would I say if he called on me?"

"Colletti!"

Colletti stood up, and in a loud voice said, "The Trapezius, sir," and sat down.

Burns went on without acknowledging the correct answer. Again, right answers were not remarkable, they were expected. I hardly heard anything over the next three hours, and I certainly couldn't read anything scribbled on the board far below. All I could do was cringe in fear of being called out in my very first moments of medical training.

Luckily for me, mine was not among the twenty or so names he did call. While I was savoring my good fortune, Dr. Burns made a cryptic announcement: each of us must make an appointment at Dr. Angel's lab. Any time will do as long as it isn't during a scheduled lecture. Dr. Angel? Upperclassmen only snickered when we asked.

I went across the street to the fraternity house, bolted down a sandwich of some sort, rushed back to the now empty pit, and read as much and as fast as I could about skin, trapezius muscle, and surrounding structures.

The combination of morgue and mortification has stayed in my head ever since, permanent reminders that real learning is a function of preparation more than review. Lesson learned.

Promptly (always promptly) at one o'clock, we filed into the dissection room where 44 bodies wrapped in thick layers of paraffin-soaked bandages were lined up on steel tables, each table with two stools on each side. It was all done alphabetically, down to the stool one was to use for the entirety of the five-month dissection process.

Ten anatomy teachers, all dressed in black wrap-around smocks, directed traffic. They were serious, efficient to a fault, and many had thick German accents. These were former German surgeons who came to the US after WWII, but because of poor or absent documentation of their training were unable to qualify for license to continue practice. Their next best option, short of leaving the profession entirely, was to become anatomy teachers. They were all about business, never exchanged banter or even pleasantries. But as teachers, they were superb.

They were also responsible for weekly anatomy tests. All 44 bodies were unwrapped just enough to tag a specific structure. Because as a group they were so fastidious, every part, no matter how minute or filamentous, was clearly visible. No tricks, either you knew it or you didn't. And woe betides the student who used a pencil to touch, lift, or move anything.

Each dissection was preceded by a detailed lecture on the exact process to be followed. Every structure from the largest muscle to the smallest nerve had to be exposed intact. Severing or pulling a nerve or blood vessel out of position was inexcusable, a disaster for all four students working on that one body.

"You're not pithing frogs anymore. Think of the corpse as your patient, and remember: you don't get a second chance in the OR."

We also learned to do everything as a team, previewing each move down to the tiniest nick before doing the actual dissection.

The body looked like a mummy from a grade B horror movie. Our first job was to turn it over and unwrap just enough of the soggy bandages to see the exact spot we were going to dissect. We began high on the back, and because so little of the body was exposed each day and the work proceeded so slowly, we didn't see the face or discover the gender for over a month.

Paradoxically, the dissection was also a race against time. No matter how well embalmed or carefully wrapped, each corpse was on an unstoppable path to decay, so considerable attention was paid to slowing down the process by limiting exposure and carefully rewrapping after each session. As fall progressed and we went deeper into the body, exposure was harder to limit, rewrapping more difficult, and tissue deterioration accelerated in unison with the olfactory assault alluded to before. And, yes, oil of wintergreen applied to a cloth mask helped considerably.

There was another, more private aspect of dissection, one we didn't talk about openly: how to cope with the reality we were going to invade and ultimately destroy the body of a man or woman who only months before had been a living person, probably a patient, someone one could easily have passed on the street. Collectively, we were initially quite respectful, no upperclassmen jokes at our table. We hoped dissection would reveal the cause of death, and we wondered if the person might have been a benevolent donor, or if this poor soul had died without anyone's notice. As fall wore on, the body began to look less and less human, more a collection of parts, each still connected in its proper place, to be studied, returned, rewrapped each day.

It's as if the person melted away leaving only a tangle of soggy parts behind. With the change, a subtle insensitivity developed in proportion to the smell and increasingly difficult tissue texture. Nicknames emerged: "Festering Fred," "Gory Gloria," and "Rottin' Robin" to name a few. It was also a way of coping with our transition to the world of medicine, a place where a lifetime of attitudes and perceptions were being turned upside down. Death used to be distant, rarely experienced close at hand. Suddenly, it was part of every day. We became indifferent to pain, particularly drawing blood from each other, or having one's partner stuff a tube down your nose into your stomach—or worse.

Embarrassment became a banished sentiment, and every needle and medical procedure became an object of learning, observed without emotional distraction.

The motto of medical students has always been: "See One, Do One, Teach One." No holding back, no fear or hesitation, and if you felt squeamish the first time you saw a procedure, believe me, that emotion was in exile the next time around.

A few weeks into the dissection, we realized our cadaver was a man, and through him, we evolved the mindset needed to move to the next step in our learning. For no particular reason I can remember, we called him Fred. In that way, we may have seemed thoughtless, but our humor was not disdainful. We looked for clues to his life, what kind of work he may have done, how he might have ended up on our dissecting table. Even today, I remember him in great detail, and still wonder about his life journey. More importantly, I remain grateful for the durable gift of his body.

I did make my appointment with Dr. Angel, having been told tauntingly by others I would be stripped naked and photographed by Dr. Angel's lovely assistant, Iris. Apparently, Dr. Angel had a grand plan to measure each and every student then and at ten-year increments forever, a project to be carried on by his trainees when he retired.[1]

When it was my turn, I found there was a lot more to it than just another snapshot. For starters, a strange physical focused mainly on endless measurements of bone length, muscle group, and skull dimensions, then blood work, and finally, yes, multiple naked pictures carefully orchestrated by Iris. Young, smiling, enjoying-it, Iris.

"Turn a little more, please. Stand straight. I want to see you straight, please." All of this while balanced on a wooden plinth, just one more unexpected knuckleball to add to the list.

The only other course for the first half of the year was Histology, parallel to gross anatomy, but on a microscopic level—and without the oil of wintergreen. It was also the foundation needed to absorb our upcoming course in Physiology, the study of the way organs, tissues, and cells operate. Together, they prepared us for Pathology, the study of disease on both the macro and microscopic levels.

---

1.   Dr. Lawrence Angel, 1915–1986; PhD from Harvard 1942; taught Biological Anthropology at Jefferson 1942–1962; then Curator of Physical Anthropology at the Smithsonian Institute until his death in 1986.

Fall gave way to winter, we finished the gross dissection, studied the brain and neuroanatomy in detail, and said goodbye to the anatomy building. The bodies were cremated in the basement morgue. We were told each body was cremated separately, that body parts were not mixed. Given the unusual care given to wrapping every tiny scrap of the body, it is highly likely that nicety was indeed observed. The fate of the ashes was not revealed, however. The anatomy building has been reborn as an upscale condo. One wonders if the tenants know the building's history.

Looking back, the excitement and challenge of learning so much so fast swamped my anxiety about how I was performing, protection that melted when I saw the details of what lay ahead in Biochemistry and Physiology, both acute reminders of professors Brinkley and Panson, and the gyrations I went through to wiggle through organic chemistry.

In college, I had time to scheme my way around a problem, and in those basic chemistry courses, math was only an occasional issue. But suddenly, the luxury of time vaporized, and math could no longer be avoided. Both courses, most especially Biochemistry, involved solving problems using calculus. And unlike college courses, these weren't transient problems to finish and forget. Quite the opposite, they were needed over and over, and retained as tools required to understand the way molecules and their compounds operate in cells and organs.

I bumped along for a while, but the reality of my situation was simply too much to ignore. I fell into a deep gloom thinking my fledgling career was about to end, defeated by my irrational phobia about numbers.

I decided it would be less humiliating to withdraw than become one of the 24 erased at the end of the year. Also, it would sell better when I applied to law school or went for a PhD in anatomy to say I withdrew when I realized medicine wasn't the path I wanted to follow. It sounded reasonable—even brave—and there would be no need to mention calculus at all.

So I went to see Dr. Cantarow, Chairman of the Department of Biochemistry, to tell him my story. I wasn't asking for anything; rather, it was simply the first step in fashioning a graceful departure.

Dr. Cantarow listened to me without expression or comment. When I finished, we sat in silence for perhaps 30 seconds before he finally spoke.

"Well, Hirsh, I'll say one thing: you've got balls."

That was not what I expected, nor was what he said next.

"You've gotten this far, you're doing well, so I'll make a deal with you. I'll personally grade all of your tests, and if you can set up the solution to the problem so I can see that if you had known the math you would have come up with the right answer, then I'll give you credit."

The deal was made, and I made it through both courses. Ironically, I had more trouble with Physiology, even though there was less math involved. Because so many had taken physiology in college, it skewed the grading scales and made me struggle harder to get even a mediocre grade.

Physiology teachers were every bit as tough as the rest. One I remember in particular was Dr. Eugene Aserinsky (1921–1998), a prickly, remote researcher who discovered the phenomenon of REM sleep. He was at Jefferson for twenty years but left in a huff when he was passed over for head of the department. He died in a car crash, the cause said to have possibly been falling asleep at the wheel.

But I survived the year, eternally grateful to Dr. Cantarow for giving me the chance to continue in spite of my math deficit. Equally, I had the support of my lab partners, each well ahead of me, especially in physiology. Best of all, there was the pleasure of upending Dr. Brinkley's prediction of failure. Still, it was a really close call, and any celebrating would have been an act of hubris, a risk I couldn't afford even with calculus in the rearview mirror.

There was very little said about disease in our first year of study, and only an occasional whiff of anything clinical—except for obstetrics. Even there, birth was seen as a natural process, not a disease, so it fit neatly into the first-year paradigm of learning about everything normal. We were assigned in rotation to obstetrical residents until each of us had seen the birth process start to finish several times.

Beyond observing births, the rotation introduced us to the many apprehensions and sudden interventions that go with even seemingly normal labor and delivery. It also introduced us to the delicate matter of examining female patients, the place our all-male culture went terribly astray. Had we been sharing wintergreen with female classmates, discussing vaginas, prostates, and more importantly, hearing their feelings and perspective on breast and pelvic examination, then the awkwardness we all felt would have been significantly reduced. More to the point, we would have been in a far better learning posture, uncomplicated by a lack of awareness of how one half of the population thinks about its interaction with the male-dominated world of clinical care.

And it wasn't just the physicians who were all-male: the professors and medical staff were also overwhelmingly male, and with that gender dominance came an attitude of male superiority, nowhere more in your face than in OB-GYN. True, there was some lip service paid to the need for discretion and professionalism in approaching the female examination, but in the end, the message was about being male, and thus in charge. The nurses—overwhelmingly female—were in on the game, too: light on empathy and heavy on the tough-it-out approach. Do what the doctor says. There was no push-back against the underlying theme of doctors in charge of a woman's reproductive health.

Though it crossed my mind that others might have similar apprehensions, I assumed the problem was mine, a lack of clinical courage based on pure ignorance. It was like being back in the line to the morgue with no clue about the anatomy of the trapezius muscle.

Happily, enormous changes over the years have significantly diminished insensitivity to women, schools now dare to address the issue openly, and an all-male obstetrical staff would be unthinkable today.

I am still grateful to the many female patients who graciously—courageously—allowed us to learn from them. It cannot have been an easy or comfortable experience.

With the first year done, we had a short, last summer break before claiming a precious seat in the pathology lab. Quite a few married at that point, I among them. Carrying on a romance was easy in college, but a considerable challenge during the first two years of medical school. There simply wasn't time. Suddenly, free time was compressed into a few precious hours on Saturday afternoon, just enough time to do a few errands and let off some steam playing inter-fraternity softball or basketball. Saturday night was also fraternity time, though alcohol was virtually invisible. Everyone was well-behaved and the place was empty well before midnight. Sunday was a full-on study day, no exceptions.

Marriage brought comfort, support, and a vivid reversal of the ennui of solitary student life. It also revived the realization there was more to life than endless study. Our wives understood the nature of our commitment and did all they could to support us.

My wife patiently studied with me, took care of most of the day-to-day chores, and never complained about being caught in the life of a medical student. She also introduced me to one of her favorite study habits, *supererogation,* the idea one should always do slightly more than one is tasked to do. If the assignment is to read three chapters, then at the very least, get a start on the fourth.

When I hit pharmacology in the second year, we were told that on tests we could use either the chemical or the trade name of a drug. Not enough, said my supererogating wife: don't settle for learning just one, know them both. It was great advice; more than that, it turned into a habit that has served me well throughout my career.

Student wives quickly found each other and shared their common mix of problems and promise. Most wives had jobs, providing needed income to support husband and sometimes family.

They also created a social web behind the daily grind, replacing the feeling of isolation with one of inclusion, cleverly using even limited time to highlight the idea that one could simultaneously study and have a life outside medicine, one with music, entertainment, and sometimes just plain good fun.

The first year was all about everything normal, the second started the focus on disease. Toward the end of year two, some basic examination skills were taught, tools needed for the next two years of training where the focus was examination, diagnosis, and treatment of disease.

The process started with Pathology and Microbiology, the fear factor strongest for the unforgiving, relentless pace of Pathology, pressed by the department chairman, Dr. Peter Herbert, and his 1,590-page textbook. In spite of its scope and complexity, we were expected to absorb the entire panoply of diseases, some quite arcane, like the study of "foreign bodies" found in various body cavities. My favorite (if one can have such a sentiment) was a paragraph on foreign bodies found in the human colon, including a toolbox containing a flashlight and a gun barrel.[2]

You might expect pathologists to be a universally somber and humorless crowd, given the nature of their work. In the operating room, for example, crucial decisions are made quickly, often based on the examination of one tiny sliver of tissue. No mistakes allowed. And they perform autopsies, often on a daily basis. That ought to dent anyone's humor.

In spite of all the warnings and apprehension fed by upperclassmen, the pathology faculty was surprisingly upbeat. The volume of material to be learned was daunting, but on the bright side: the playing field was suddenly level. The boys from Villanova and Marshall had not taken undergraduate pathology.

Microbiology was an entirely different matter, not because of the subject, but because of the man who almost single-handedly ran the department. In fact, I can't remember the name of a single

2. Page 954 of Herbut's *Pathology*, 1958 edition.

teacher in microbiology other than the boss, known by his initials, "K.G."

Again, upperclassmen gleefully told us we were in for a shock when we met K.G.

On the first day, after a benign, no-grilling opening lecture, we went to the laboratory to find our workstation. For the first time, nothing was alphabetical, but as we quickly learned, what seemed like a random assignment of places was actually a well-calculated plan directed by K.G.'s invisible and inscrutable planning.

We were directed to stand at our places while K.G. went about meeting and talking to each of us individually, a process that absorbed the entire afternoon. While waiting our turn, we could study, but nothing else, not even talk. Clearly, the entire time was devoted to being sized up by K.G. I didn't have long to wait as my spot was the second one in the front of the lab.

K.G. stood in front of me, literally looked me over, consulted a small notebook, then spoke.

"Hirsh." Pause. "Andover and Yale. No doctors in your family, right?"

"Correct, sir," I answered, wondering where this was headed.

"Your father is an engineer. No points off for that." Another pause, then he snapped the book shut and said, "Keep your eyes open, Hirsh. And two points off your final grade for Yale."

That was it. And so it went for the rest of the afternoon, one by one, each of us had the same experience. Eerily, K.G. seemed to know everyone's background, at least the parts about schools attended and parents' occupation. Almost everyone lost a point or more for something. Ivy League schools: two points off. Even some non-Ivy League schools cost points—for some even more obscure reason. Either parent a physician? Another point off for each. Only graduate education before medical school netted an added point.

The reason for K.G.'s well-advertised eccentricities was unknown.

Upperclassmen said he was an embittered man teaching a profession he held in disdain, allegedly because of the introduction of penicillin in the 1940s, an innovation that overnight cancelled K.G.'s life work: a system of using an anti-serum for the treatment of pneumococcal pneumonia, a common and often deadly form of the disease. Like many scientists in the first half of the twentieth century, K.G. had been searching for a method to treat infection, a seemingly impossible task. In the days before sulfa and penicillin, a tiny scratch could become infected and lead to death. An infected tooth, boil, or tonsillitis could kill you outright, unthinkable in today's world. K.G.'s work could have put him on the path to fame, glory, and comfort, but when his dream was torpedoed by penicillin, he gave up his research and turned to teaching. Penicillin came into general use in 1944, K.G. joined the Jefferson faculty in 1946. He retired in June 1967 and died suddenly two months later.

Just how much truth there was in the legend of the eccentric genius I can't say. But one fact I can add with complete certainty: K.G. sought and obtained the appointment of Jefferson's first full-time female professor.

His motivation was obscure, but there was no doubt about what we were in for: there would be no such thing as anonymity in his world. K.G. had his own system, starting with never forgetting a student's name or how he was doing in class. He had his own idea of what a level playing field looked like, and surprise could come from any direction.

The surprise factor didn't take long to show itself. A few days into our work, we were tested on our newly acquired specimen staining technique, the all-important method of using dyes to make an organism's structure visible under the microscope. Without a stain, identification is virtually impossible.

The test was simple enough: at each place, a glass slide with an unstained specimen was parked on a piece of white paper. One had to stain it, look at the results under the microscope, and identify the bacterium. One slide, one stain, one answer.

I applied the proper stain, let it set, washed off the excess, put it under the microscope and looked...at nothing. The field was empty, and there was nothing I could do to bring it back. I took a guess, turned in my answer, and on the way out the door, K.G. said, "I told you to keep your eyes open, Hirsh." The specimen had been placed on the *underside* of the slide, not the top, and unless one looked to see which side it was on, one would make the fatal mistake of staining an empty space and washing away the sample.

Ouch. Another lesson learned.

Another trick we were warned about was the finger-in-the-urine gambit, an apocryphal tale every medical student knew but never actually saw. According to the story, the instructor would hold up two flasks of urine, one said to be from a diabetic patient, the other from a non-diabetic. The diabetic's urine would contain sugar which, it was said, could be detected by taste. The instructor would plunge a finger into the first flask, taste it, then repeat the performance with the second flask. Then the flasks were passed around for the students to taste and compare, and finally say, which was the diabetic's urine.

After a lot of gagging, the instructor would say the entire group had failed, because both samples were the same. The *real* purpose of the demonstration was to teach observation skills. Then he would repeat his show in slow motion. He carefully inserted his index finger into the flask, withdrew, and folded the finger into his palm while he inserted his second, unsullied, finger into his mouth. It may have happened in 1891, but happily, not in 1961.

Along with tricks to sharpen observational skills, K.G. was known for his small-group quiz sessions, a major factor in one's final grade. Forty or so of us would gather, K.G. at the front consulting and making notes in his ever-present little black book. Following an invisible script, over the ensuing three hours each of us would be asked three, sometimes four, questions. Each question was short and had only one right answer. Right to the point, straight up or down, no wiggle room.

Strangely, I came to look forward to the sessions. Normally, I hate being called out, but the Yale penalty was stuck in my crop, fueling my determination never to get tripped up by the enigmatic professor. And even though I knew perfectly well I was being manipulated into a mental arm-wrestling match, I couldn't resist the challenge to push myself. Unlike the Brinkley crush, this time anger was displaced by determination to learn—a far healthier and durable motivation.

I did well in the course, watched my average carefully, and sure enough: at the end, K.G. knocked two points off my final grade. I knew he would, but somehow I didn't mind.

The second half of the year brought us to the leading edge of medical practice, starting with the fundamentals of taking a medical history and doing a physical exam. This was the moment when we began to separate normal from abnormal, give it a name, and begin to think about what to do with the results.

Learning the questions needed for even the most basic history was awkward and halting at first, far from the seamless alignment needed to allow one to track the process from a single complaint to a working diagnostic hypothesis. I had 3x5 cards in my pocket covered with questions written in tiny letters, all in the right order, plus a helpful set of mnemonics—anything to keep up the flow of information. Interns and residents made it look so easy, like a musician who has mastered an instrument, constant repetition allowed them to follow an invisible path effortlessly through myriad questions to arrive at a diagnosis. I counted the number of standard questions in a complete history of an otherwise healthy adult with a straightforward illness. The number is 241. Try that with a two-page questionnaire.

It slowly dawned on me that trying to memorize it all was getting in the way. The history is really a song with a title, "Chief Complaint," supported by a rhythm carrying the investigation along a logical pathway, each note a refinement of the one before, each verse a complete idea, all the way to the last chorus, the "Diagnostic Impression."

Through weeks of practice, I came to rely less on Q-cards and more on the feeling I could begin to follow the breadcrumbs all the way through. No matter how long or short, the history always broke down into three separate, specific zones. Adhering to the sequence, listening carefully to the patient's words, and fashioning the next question out of the last answer served as an unfailing guide to a proposed diagnosis, one that could be defended with hard data gathered from the complete history.

The very first part of the history, no matter what the specialty, is the Chief Complaint (CC) and Reason for Admission (or Evaluation, or Consultation, depending on the circumstances). It is recorded in the patient's exact words—always in quotes—followed by an even shorter statement of duration saying exactly how long the problem has been present. Nothing else is said in the Chief Complaint. It is the starting point, the title of the song. All the verses to follow are designed to explain the meaning of the title.

The first verse after the Chief Complaint is the History of the Present Illness (HPI), and its big question is: Why Now? Nothing moves forward until it is clear why the patient is here today as opposed to last week or even yesterday. The HPI tells you what is new, separating it from past history—even within events in the same disease recurring over time. Each episode is treated differently, almost like a separate disease. It also helps you see how the patient understands and copes with the problem. Even in the most chronic conditions, there is always something that distinguishes the current situation from the same problem days or weeks before. Getting at that issue is the key to diagnosis and management. It also helps the patient better understand the illness. Patients who have that knowledge participate more effectively in treatment.

The next verse is Past Medical History (PMH), the search for material that supports and explains the emergence of the patient's current problem. There is a slight variation in the psychiatric history: the Past Medical History becomes the Past Psychiatric History, the Past Medical History is moved further into the process.

Next, is the Family History (FH), important because so many illnesses are heritable. Symptoms that don't seem to hang together can suddenly be explained learning a relative has had a similar condition the patient might never have thought could be connected. Also, a vital key to treatment is knowing what medications may have worked (or failed) for family members. A solid treatment rule is "When in doubt, reach first for the one with the best record among blood relatives."

More verses follow covering relationship history, habits (like drug, smoking, and alcohol use), and just before the Diagnostic Impression, the hugely important and detailed Mental Status Examination (MSE), starting with simple observations about handedness, dress, hygiene, walking, use of language, affect (feeling tone heard in voice, pace of speech, and inflection) and cognitive state. Psychiatric and neurological mental status examination is more detailed, but follows the same basic vector: what light does the patient's thinking and behavior *right this minute* throw on the diagnostic possibilities?

Next, a Diagnostic Impression is made along with "Rule-Outs," other possibilities that must be explained to support or change the final diagnosis. That takes one to the final chorus: Recommendations, the plan for suggestions of further diagnostic evaluation and treatment.

The first time I took a complete history by myself, unobserved, was on a neurology ward. I remember the patient quite well, and would love to break the rules to use his name in appreciation for being so gracious with my bumbling attempt to gather a coherent history. But on the off-off chance a relative might take offense, I'll simply say, "Thanks," and add his name under my breath.

He was an elderly man who had suffered a mild stroke, leaving him partly paralyzed on one side, and it affected his speech—the part that bothered him the most. My task was to take the history, focus heavily on the mental status, read the results of his physical exam, and be ready to come up with a coherent statement about diagnosis.

I made a terrible mess of the questions, became tangled in the sequence, distracted by the man's problems with speech. Clearly, he sensed my struggle, and rather than be resentful or impatient, he made an enormous attempt to speak clearly. He even filled in some of the gaps with what he had heard other doctors say about his condition. When I was quizzed about the examination, it was clear I barely knew what I was up to, but thanks to the patient's tutelage, I was at least able to proffer a ballpark diagnosis. It also gave me enough to make a good guess about which cranial artery may have been involved. You can see why I remain in debt to this generous man.

Good history taking is still an art, and cannot be done with a computer program or check list. But time is everything today, reliance on computer algorithms and checklists is a fact of life, all of which argues that as patients we must be assertive in explaining our problem, not letting go until we feel the physician understands our concerns. A good rule of thumb is to remember the pivotal separation between "Why Now?" and everything that has come before. Don't let the physician press on until you feel you have said as much as possible about exactly why you are in his office at that moment.

Today's medical students don't fully master the details needed to take a comprehensive history, or appreciate the fact it is literally part of the physical examination. Interviews simply can't be complete rushing through a computer-driven program. Observing basics like handedness, facial expression, body movement, and a host of other subtle observables is needed to perform a *complete* physical examination.

No surprise, the core issue stressed from the start in both the history and physical examination is *observation*. K.G. was absolutely right: the key to everything depends on keeping your eyes open right from the first moment you see the patient.

It doesn't work that way today. Think about it: the last time you went to see a physician, after doing battle with all the insurance, consent, and HIPPA forms, you filled out a symptom check list. Little boxes, just yes or no. Then someone weighed you, took your blood pressure through your shirt using an automated pressure cuff, parked you in a tiny office, and left.

When the doctor arrived, he was carrying a laptop computer, said a pleasant hello, turned his attention to the computer screen, and asked what brought you in today in order to capture the Chief Complaint and Reason for Evaluation. You were aware of time pressure, so chances are you had rehearsed your statement to keep it short, resisting the urge to speak about any other problems bothering you.

Sometimes there is no physical at all, but if there is, it will be short and limited to the jurisdiction of your Chief Complaint, a time saver but enough to satisfy the minimum the insurance company demands to justify the cost of your visit. Next, a flurry of typing, possibly following an algorithm of diagnostic and treatment possibilities; finally, discussion of testing and possible referral, followed by a prescription emailed to your pharmacy. Side effect issues are covered in a *Reader's Digest* review, there is another handshake, and you're done. See you in a month.

There is a high probability you would have been referred to another physician for further diagnostic work and treatment. It's an easy move to make, covers the clinician's tail, and gives you the reassuring feeling everyone is focused on your care.

Trouble is, it doesn't work that way in real life. The speed and abbreviated nature of your primary care visit leaves gaps and uncertainties to be fixed by the second physician. Spread the responsibility and move on to the next case. You might also expect the physician to pick up the phone and explain the situation to the next doctor. Or that the wonders of the electronic record would instantly make everything available to the new clinician; equally, the results of the consultation visit would zoom back to your primary care doctor, then on to you.

The phone call doesn't happen because the PCP is pressed for time, doesn't get paid to make phone calls, and time out for unpaid labor is frowned on by the office manager. Also, there is a high probability the two physicians don't even know each other, especially in urban settings. The system invites abuse because it's all about moving along quickly, every step guided by the computer, each step designed to minimize liability and maximize revenue. Combining the large number of patients to be seen with the complexity of the larger medical system means this is probably the best you'll get.

We were also taught that when doing a consultation, it was mandatory to write a letter to the referring physician, always starting with:

"Dear Dr. Jones, Thank you referring your patient, Mr. Smith…"

The key word is "Your." You sent the note promptly, thus assuring the timely arrival of referral information. It was fast, polite, and not even attempted today in spite of the fact such a letter could be dispatched through the internet. Oops. Not so fast: computer systems in the two offices don't talk to each other. The referral document will have to get there some other way. Usually, it is handed to you to be presented to the consultant at the time of your appointment. Unfortunately, that means the consultant will not have been able to preview it and prepare before the visit. Most consults are straightforward, so it doesn't make much difference. Add complexity, however, and time compression becomes a greater disadvantage.

After you see the consultant, a clinical note is sent back to the referring PCP. All too often, it doesn't get there in time for your follow-up PCP visit. The doctor tells the nurse, the nurse tells the secretary who calls the other office to request a FAX, but that can't be done until they check for a proper release of information, and so on. Ever been in that predicament?

Lamenting the loss of the older system is a waste of time. We are not going back to some idealized time when individual care carried the day. That's gone, and we now have a system that isn't really a system at all. It's a collection of systems, no two exactly alike or following the same set of rules. It has also become political, people choosing up sides to defend one model over another. Because it's so political, truth and fiction are mangled in a way that proves my idea is better than yours. And it's not just here in the USA, it's everywhere. No two countries have the same system or set of rules everyone lives with. To the extent people think about what other countries do, we tend to assume that everyone else has a single payer system, that ours is the only free, unfettered, market-driven form of health care around. The truth is, while the proportions vary, insurance and government systems run side by side in almost all economies.

But back in the early 1960s when I was stumbling along, it was all about the patient, not the system. The system was you, and it was up to you to learn the science and techniques that would result in the best care possible. Responsible practice was self-generated, not defined by insurance companies or office managers.

The stumble factor increased exponentially for all of us as we began to learn the techniques of the physical examination at the end of the second year. Our first patients were, of course, each other. But we were used to it. We had been taking each other's blood for months, I had twice had a nasogastric tube threaded through my nose into my stomach, so the idea we were now going to strip down and examine each other in a class was not the least bit daunting. And Iris wasn't there.

There were many rotations that year, some like Dermatology, Radiology, and Psychiatry fairly short, others like Surgery, Internal Medicine, and OB-GYN longer because each of those had separate subspecialties. Dermatology was bewildering because every skin problem looked like the last one, but I did come away with two lasting principles, one sorta true, the other vital. First, there is an overarching adage concerning the treatment of skin disorders: If it's wet—dry it. If it's dry—wet it. If that fails, use a steroid. The more serious is a cautionary reminder: The skin is the body's largest sensory organ, often the first place to signal the presence of an underlying or emerging illness. Dismiss the rule at your peril. I would add that a similar caution comes from the part of the body most disregarded by physicians: the teeth. A tiny infection at the root of a tooth, sometimes barely felt, can seed the bloodstream with an infection that if unrecognized and untreated, may have grave consequences, either as a subtle infection in the brain, heart valves, or an explosive infection in another organ.

Pediatrics was a different experience altogether, primary because the majority of patients were healthy, and it was our job to see to it they stayed that way. Also, it was a specialty with a roughly equal balance of male and female clinicians. That did not, however, translate into the department head being a woman. Far from it, the Chief was straight out of the abrasive teaching school. Like so many others of his ilk, he seemed to delight in berating students who failed to answer one of his zinger questions. I was used to it, but still watched in fear, knowing it would inevitably be my turn to be scorched. Finally, it came: a curve ball question about physiology, not one about disease. What happens in aspirin overdose, and where does the non-metabolized aspirin go?

I knew better than try to work gracefully through the multiple steps, especially when it came to explaining the role of the kidney. Rather than look the fool, I decided it was better to take the heat up front.

"Sir, I only know that it causes a state of hyper-metabolism, potassium and sodium drop, and beyond that, I'm lost."

The Chief looked at me for a long five seconds while I stood waiting for the blast.

"Well! Finally, an honest man."

I was stunned, and more than a little relieved. After that, the questions seemed less hostile, and I relaxed, studied harder, and later, got up the courage to ask if he would become our child's pediatrician. He accepted.

While 90% of the time it was a pleasant rotation, there were inevitably wrenching moments when things went terribly wrong.

Childhood leukemia was fundamentally untreatable, as were diseases like cystic fibrosis, some seizure disorders, severe asthma, and many more. Dealing with the death of a child right before your eyes is impossible to accept and process emotionally. Oncologists have a special ability to work in this minefield. They are quick to remind us that the diseases we can now treat successfully are many, that treatment today is far more hopeful than even a decade ago. Cure rates for acute lymphocytic leukemia, for example, now approach 80%, unheard of when I was in training.

One case that still haunts me involved a boy about ten who had heart disease. An accumulation of fluid in the sack surrounding his heart was putting deadly pressure on his heart. The only way to relieve the pressure was to insert a needle and draw off the fluid. I was assigned the job of holding the boy in a sitting position while the resident inserted the needle. Seconds into that procedure the boy went limp and literally died in my arms. I was stunned, and barely heard the resident tell me to go to the waiting room and tell his parents their son had died. The resident and his group left, and I had no other way out.

Together with a nurse, we broke the news. It was beyond awful, and I'll never really be able to get rid of the vivid image of the boy, and the moment we told the parents what had happened. Perhaps the strangest moment, however, came as I struggled to keep my emotions in check and provide some tiny shred of support. The boy's father put his hand on my shoulder and said, "It's not your fault." How do some people manage such grace in the midst of their own despair?

Similar moments followed in other clinics: the woman in normal labor who suddenly suffered a devastating stroke caused by a rare leakage of amniotic fluid into her bloodstream, the patient who committed suicide in his bed by cutting his wrist, found by a nurse in the morning lying in a huge pool of blood. And it wasn't always patients. A pathology resident in the staff dining room almost casually said, "I just ruptured an aneurism, I can feel it trickling," and fell over dead. Or the time I was sitting with a small group of residents talking while waiting for a professor to appear when one suddenly said, "God! I feel weird." He died on the spot—another aneurism.

But it wasn't all grim. I was assigned to my first ER experience in a Camden, New Jersey, hospital—my job simply was to watch and learn. Most of the first day was quiet, sometimes with no patients at all, a chance to sit with the staff, drink coffee, and feel on the edge of inclusion. Suddenly, we heard a police siren clearly heading our way. Everyone jumped up, ready for whatever came next. The siren died, replaced by the wailing of a female voice. The door burst open: two policemen made way for a woman holding a bath towel around the hand of a youngster perhaps five years old. The kid was calm, but his mother was frantic.

"My child has been bitten by a SNAKE!" she screamed. "Do something!!"

A snake? In Camden? I know a lot about snakes, always liked them, and I knew the only dangerous possibility was a copperhead bite, rare, but not impossible. The wailing continued as the child was lifted onto a gurney, and the nurse started to unwrap the towel. The child watched, more interested than alarmed. As the last fold of the towel came off, the snake jumped out, fell on the floor and started a furious wriggle, unable to get any traction on the tile floor.

Everyone ran out of the room: the cops, the nurse, the ER doctor—and the mother. That left the boy, me, and the garter snake. I picked up the snake letting it slide through my hands in an endless journey to nowhere. The others watched from the door. I showed the snake to the boy, let him touch it, and took the poor creature out to a grassy area behind the hospital. The tiny bite was cleansed, he got a tetanus shot, and they left.

In another ER, this one in a rough section of Philadelphia where we saw a lot of trauma, I very quickly learned about wound care and suturing. On one particularly busy evening, a man came in with an enormous foot wound. Somehow, he had sliced the area between his big toe and the second toe. Looking at it, I wondered how the intern was going to approach it. A simple cut would only require simple stitching, something I had already done many times, but dealing with a wound like this was entirely different. If not done properly, the patient might never walk a straight line again.

The intern was very busy, and after looking at the wound, turned to me and said, "Clean it, close it." I said something like, "Are you kidding?" He said it is really quite simple, and rattled off what to close first with what type of suture, and left. Okay, this is it. I did it, terrified I wouldn't get the sequence right. The man left, and I still wonder if he walks with a limp.

I also got my first taste of the interaction of police and unruly suspects, often men and women feigning grievous injury as a way to delay or even dodge incarceration. I had never before come face-to-face with violence, or the stunning lengths criminals go to manipulate, intimidate, and literally threaten anyone trying to deal with them, especially when they were drunk or high on heroin. At times, it was literally frightening, and it wasn't always just the crooks who were scary. The cops were used to it, usually restrained, but sometimes it was simply too much even for them.

One late night, the police brought in a particularly menacing, intoxicated man to be examined before they took him to jail, not so much out of concern he might be in some way injured, but because if he sobered up and had a real injury, they would have to bring him back—twice the hassle. Prevention is always better than added paperwork.

Examining the man was impossible, even when the cops held him down. The intern suggested sedation even though it was risky in a patient with an unknown substance—or substances—on board. The cops said they had a better idea, took the handcuffed man back to the paddy wagon, pushed him into the back, shut the door, shot down the driveway about thirty yards, and slammed on the brakes. They backed up and did it again. When they dragged the dazed man back into the ER, it was relatively easy to do a cursory exam and send them all on their way.[3]

---

3. There are two theories about how police transport vehicles acquired the name "Paddy Wagons." The first comes from the fact the Irish made up a disproportionate number of police in the late 19th and early 20th centuries. "Paddy" was a prejudicially shortened version of Patrick, like

At that same ER, I was tasked with examining a hulking, menacing-looking man, handcuffed, who was pinned between two cops doing their best to keep him from squirming. He grunted and growled but wouldn't answer any questions. In fact, he wouldn't say a word.

"Open your mouth," I said.

He clenched his jaw and stared at me.

"Open your f...ing mouth," said one of cops.

No response. The cop looked around, and while seemingly looking at something across the room, gave the man a hard shot to the stomach. His mouth popped open, and a spit-coated, wadded one-hundred-dollar bill popped out.

The man looked at me and said, "If you hadn't said anything, I would have split it with you." Sure.

Another brush with reality in that same ER started as what seemed like a relatively easy case. A young woman was brought in with right lower abdominal pain, an examination quickly revealing the obvious fact she had acute appendicitis, demanding immediate surgery. The surgical resident was called, and I was told to go along to hold retractors and observe the operation. In what I foolishly thought to be a reassuring gesture to her parents, I said as we left for the OR, "Don't worry, we'll take good care of your daughter," to which her father responded angrily, "You'd better, or I'll sue the hell out of you!"

Another, more common anomaly in down-and-out parts of the city was methanol poisoning caused by drinking "Squeeze." Methanol, also called wood alcohol and denatured alcohol, is a close cousin of ethanol, the essence of all alcoholic beverages,

---

"Mick," from Michael. The other theory dates first use to the Civil War. In 1863, there were riots in New York over a new draft law, one that swept up a disproportionate number of the poor, mostly Irish people. The wealthy could legally avoid the draft by either paying someone to take their place, or simply paying a $3,000 fee. For the poor, there was no option but to be hauled off to war in a Paddy wagon.

a simple molecule with literally thousands of applications in medicine and industry. You can poison yourself acutely with recreational alcohol (ethanol), but it takes a lot to threaten your life. Methanol, on the other hand, is a potent poison. A single ounce can kill, and relatively small amounts can cause disorientation, loss of consciousness, and blindness. It has a pungent smell and vile taste, thus the perfect thing to add to products containing ethanol to keep people from drinking it accidentally—or on purpose.

When homeless people couldn't get cheap booze or wine, they sometimes turned in desperation to Sterno, a cheap gelatinous product invented in 1900 by Mr. Sterneau to warm his copper chafing dishes. It contains both ethanol and methanol, and because the methanol doesn't destroy it's cousin, it's possible to get hammered by squeezing the jelly through a stocking, mixing it with Royal Crown Cola—and drinking it. "R.C." was the essential additive, said to subdue the rancid taste enough to get it down.

We saw several cases of Squeeze poisoning, usually about 10–12 hours after drinking it when the symptoms accelerated. Treatment was "supportive," meaning support breathing, hydration, and correcting high levels of acidity in the blood. Many were left with fried retinas, dementia, and kidney failure.

While deliberate use is a rarity in the United States today, methanol poisoning is still prevalent in underdeveloped countries. In India, in February 2019, a batch of contaminated bootleg liquor killed 95 people and sickened hundreds more. The combination of desperation and greed prevailed in spite of the fact that "it smelled like diesel fuel and looked unusually milky."

ERs are a great place to learn about life in the real world.

Our introduction to Internal Medicine, while refreshingly non-confrontational, was a challenging tour of its many specialty parts: cardiology, endocrinology (hormone disorders like thyroid disease), gastroenterology (the gut and liver), hematology (blood disease, anemia), infectious disease, nephrology (kidney), and rheumatology (joints).

In each, the emphasis was on the specifics of history taking, physical examination, and interpretation of lab and testing results. It was here we started examining people other than lab partners. We also learned the basics of drawing blood under any circumstance and starting IVs with the correct fluids, both fundamental skills to be mastered ahead of senior year and internship.

Neurology and Psychiatry were similarly calm, especially neurology, the John le Carre specialty: find the hidden diagnosis by following clues weaving in and out of various brain, spinal, and nerve pathways. Which one explains the symptoms? Which are dead ends? Which tiny finding will take you to the culprit? It was a brain game in every sense of the word.

Psychiatry was totally confusing. The textbook was dry as a Chilean desert, filled with arcane ideas about suppressed memory, sexual innuendo, and alleged "dynamic" explanations supporting a diagnosis about which there was often absolutely nothing to be done. It all smacked of Freud, psychoanalysis, and other falderal none of us took to be part of mainstream medicine.

Only a decade before we began our training, psychiatric treatments were scant and scary. One example: insulin coma treatment, cooked up in 1927, based on the erroneous idea that epileptics were protected from developing schizophrenia because they had seizures. Insulin was injected to drive blood sugar down until the patient experienced a seizure. The perilous procedure lasted into the early 1950s. Later, electrical current replaced insulin to induce seizures. Known variously as "shock therapy," electroconvulsive therapy or ECT, it came into use in the late 1930s in Europe, and in 1940 in the United States. It was dramatically safer than insulin coma, but controversial from the start—and remains so in spite of many refinements and long and successful use.

In 1935, Antonio Moniz introduced the lobotomy as a treatment for patients with severe psychosis, principally schizophrenia. It was a draconian procedure done with a modified icepick called a "leucotome"; a later, improved model was called the "orbitoclast." The device was thrust past the eyeball into the brain, swept back

and forth, and withdrawn. It became a mainstream treatment, felt
to be successful because it produced varying degrees of robotic
tranquility. Moniz received the Nobel Prize for Medicine in 1949,
and while he is long forgotten, his treatment—like insulin coma—
lasted until 1951, and the pejorative term "lobotomy" lingers in
the popular lexicon.

To us, the few drugs available to treat mental illness were
poorly understood and freighted with side effects—all of it beyond
our grip at that point. Treatment was still largely based on psychoanalytic principles, a learning black hole, largely dismissed by
most of the medical faculty. Our clinical experience was almost
cynical: we were taken to a state hospital to be shown a group of
delusional people literally paraded into an auditorium and encouraged to talk about their wild ideas. There really were people who
thought they were Jesus Christ or Napoleon, the tragedy of their
plight lost in the circus atmosphere. Clearly, it was entertainment—not teaching.

What we should have been taught was that hopeless confinement in state hospitals was on the way out, yielding to a sea-change
in treatment ushered in with the introduction of early versions
of truly effective psychiatric medication. Part of the reason we
were kept in the dark even ten years into the process, was a battle
that raged between the stubborn analytic group in charge of the
profession, and an evolving group of scientists who realized the
future of treatment lay in understanding brain chemistry to find
drugs with targeted actions, pinpoint chemical intervention to
lessen or even reverse some forms of mental illness, especially
schizophrenia, depression, and anxiety disorders.

The revolution we didn't appreciate began at 10:00 a.m. on
January 19, 1952, at the Salpetrie Hospital in Paris, when a patient,
Jacques Lh., was given the first-ever dose of Thorazine. Discovered by a chemist, and administered by a surgeon, it really was
literally the moment modern psychiatric treatment began. The
improvement was both instant and dramatic. News spread, and
in the spring of that year, the head of Smith, Kline & French

pharmaceutical laboratories in Philadelphia brought a vial of the magic substance back from Europe in his pocket.

"Anything to declare, sir?"

"No, nothing."

By mid-May, SKF was producing Thorazine with spectacular results. By the end of the decade, the number of patients confined in snake pit mental hospitals dropped in half, and many closed their rusty gates permanently. Thorazine was followed by more refined drugs, accelerating the pace of treatment options for people with crippling psychosis. Antidepressants started to trickle in by the late 1950s, but we were still only getting a toehold in how to use them. Valium showed up in 1963—a smash hit drug, itself followed by a trail of other antianxiety medications, though it took a while to recognize their potential for abuse.

At a 1989 conference on psychiatric milestones, as I was about to introduce the key developer of Valium, Sir Malcolm Lader, I said to him, "It is a great honor to be able to introduce the man who brought us such a revolutionary drug."

"I wish to hell I'd never heard of it," he snapped, obviously aware and disturbed by the drug's addictive properties. I would quickly add, however, that it is indeed an important medication, has many uses, and like many with habituating potential, it is not the drug as much as sloppy prescribing that is responsible for its problems. Addiction isn't instant, but takes months of poorly monitored use to begin to cause problems. Part of proper prescribing involves knowing one's patient well enough to find non-habituating substitutes for those predisposed to addiction. Sometimes, there simply isn't an effective substitute; in those cases, frank discussion, tight control of each prescription, and a rigid discontinuation plan will give the patient needed relief without adding addiction to his problems.

There was another enormous change happening in 1963, one it's safe to say none of us knew or cared about: the start of a national effort to bring meaningful mental health care to everyone, not just the few warming their buns on the analytic couch.

Freud—let's give him credit for this one—wrote in a letter in the mid-1930s as he approached the end of his life, that in the future, the cure for severe mental illness would come from chemists, not analysts. Further, he predicted that only "neurosis," presumably anything short of psychosis, would remain the purview of psychiatrists, but given the enormous number of people with some form of mental illness coupled with obvious limitations in the time and expense (and throw in effectiveness) of analysis, an entirely new system of treatment would be needed. He suggested a community system, a pyramid with psychiatrists at the top supervising expanding layers of psychologists, social workers, and ancillary specialists below.

A near exact system was suggested by New York Congressman Jack Ewalt in 1963, taken up by President Kennedy, and became the Community Mental Health system we have today. Remember, too, that better medications, along with an expanding sense of how to support the recovery of patients with counseling, social services, and a host of other modalities, made the community system possible.

So much for psychiatry in my third and fourth years: an understanding of diagnosis, some timid acquaintance with medication, and not much else.

With the start of the third year, the first National Board examination was behind us, and we were ready to start applying basic medical science to the reality of clinical care. The transition was dramatic, starting with my first official pharmaceutical industry bribe: a black doctor's bag containing a stethoscope, ophthalmoscope, and a blood pressure cuff. The ophthalmoscope easily converted to an otoscope, both hand-held mini versions of the microscope allowing instant evaluation of a patient's eyes and ears. The ophthalmoscope allows one to look into the eyeball, revealing the mars-colored landscape of the retina with its tiny, thread-like blood vessels, and a clear view of the optic nerve as it enters the back of eye, just a few millimeters from the brain itself. There is no other place in the human body where you can see a naked, functioning nerve, artery, or vein, a picture instantly revealing a storehouse of information about health and disease.

The view through an otoscope—looking into the ear at the eardrum—though vital for ear and balance issues, isn't nearly as breathtaking as looking at the retina, especially when all one sees is a wall of earwax.

I felt like the sheriff with a new pair of six guns as I walked around with my bag of authenticating tools. For the first time, I could relax a bit, let go of the idea I would get ambushed by a math problem I couldn't solve or a chemistry question I couldn't answer. No, from then on it was clinical science, new, fascinating, and reachable. Take that, Brinkley!

Though there were many exceptions, the third year was generally the "See One" year. Most "Do One" experiences were reserved for the fourth year, preparation for the internship to follow. It also dawned on me that unless I was run over by a chart rack, I could have my license to practice medicine in three years. Now it was time to start thinking about what direction I might take at that magical point in my career.

Ooops! Hubris was creeping in, the mistake of thinking of specialty before I found out about aptitude, what I was really capable of doing well in a sustained way. I still had no real idea about each specialty, and no business getting ahead of myself. Still, when people asked what I intended to do, I answered, "Surgery." It sounded good, but was a bad mistake, as I would soon find out.

The plan for the third year was about sampling and being tested repeatedly in all specialties and their subdivisions. While some of my fellow students genuinely did have a bead on where they wanted to go, most of us were still feeling our way along, waiting for the call.

My first major "Do One" came early in the third year, an exception to the rule thrust on me from a completely unexpected direction. My wife was pregnant, and her care, like the care of all medical students' wives, was provided *pro bono* by members of the OB-GYN faculty. That included all of the hospital costs associated with the delivery, and any other care that might be required post-delivery for mother and child. Some members of the staff were more popular than others, largely because of their affable, less-confrontational teaching style, and we counted ourselves lucky to be accepted by the most sought-after of the faculty group.

My wife got the obstetrician she wanted, although rotation within the clinician's group meant there was no guarantee he (always a "he") would actually be there for the delivery. Her labor was long, and in those days delivery was handled in a way that would be considered heresy today, largely because analgesia during labor was scant at best, and anything smacking of "natural childbirth" was considered a naive oddity to be discouraged. In reality, decisions about labor were less about the mother and more a function of staff convenience. "Natural childbirth" brought with it an element of uncertainty, a challenge to the authority of the OB staff. The strong-willed nurses were no help either. They were the enforcers of the system. Uppity women were not welcome in their ranks or as patients.

Because it was feared a patient might impulsively reach an ungloved hand into the sterile sheets, her hands were shackled to the table with wrist restraints. Her labor continued without much in the way of analgesia, then at the last moment, as the birth was finally starting, she was knocked out, not only missing the birth, but allowing the physician to apply forceps, do an episiotomy (incision to enlarge the birth canal), all without alerting the patient to any of it. Hey! Wake up, here's your baby, those stitches will soon heal. You won't hear it today, but the last stitch placed in the episiotomy repair was called the "husband stitch," since it retightened the vagina after childbirth.

An alternative to being snowed with anesthetics at the last minute was the dreaded spinal anesthesia. The procedure was difficult to tolerate at any time, but especially so during the final moments of labor, and could not be given earlier because along with stopping pain, it also it stopped labor. That meant several things, starting with the need to get the baby delivered quickly by mechanical means—forceps again. It also left the patient paralyzed below the waist for several hours, often with a vicious headache thrown in for good measure.

The epidural, so easily given earlier in labor without interfering with its progress, was a novelty, not part of the picture until 1970. Technically, it is quite different from spinal anesthesia. Here's a brief explanation of why: There are two separate membranes surrounding the spine itself. The "spinal" means the needle penetrates both membranes into the fluid area around the spine. The "epidural" stops short of the second membrane containing the spine. It puts anesthetic in the area between the two membranes, numbing pain nerves without causing paralysis.

Today, the epidural is routine, a splendid way to moderate the pain of labor allowing the mother to make clear-headed decisions while fully experiencing the birth of her child, all without suffering paralysis or headache afterward.

Another enormous change is the fact that today the father is routinely invited into the delivery room, a rarity before the early 1980s. Husbands paced around a waiting room smoking cigarettes anxiously waiting for the obstetrician to make his entrance to announce grandly that he had delivered the baby, and pretty soon—after the mother was awake—the grateful husband would be allowed to see his wife and child.

Because I was a medical student, it was expected I would be present, always the chance to learn, not a function of family togetherness. In our situation, as the birth began, the obstetrician said, "You've been here a while, step up and deliver this baby." I had witnessed deliveries, but never come close to taking part. But there was no backing out, that would have been unheard of, so I did step up and caught our son as he emerged. By the way, my role didn't end with the delivery of the child. There was an umbilical cord and placenta to reckon with. I demurred on the episiotomy repair. My wife was snowed, had no idea what was going on, and was somewhere between surprised and shocked when she heard what had happened.

The OB-GYN rotation was divided between tangential participation in delivering babies, holding retractors during cesarean and GYN surgery, and OB-GYN outpatient clinic work. But it all began with learning how to do a pelvic examination, something we had seen many times but never actually performed.

It was presented entirely in technical terms, the focus on technique, especially the tricky part of being able to feel the ovaries through the vaginal wall. Again, it was all male, all technical, without anything beyond a perfunctory nod in the direction of respecting privacy. Since the pelvic exam was a fact of life, there was no attempt in the learning phase to help ease the apprehension of a shy or naïve patient.

When it came to the examination itself, a patient was recruited from the clinic population. Clinics at that time served surrounding neighborhoods, providing care at no cost, the pro quo being an understanding that in every sense of the word, care was also a teaching/learning experience for medical students. When it was time for our initial chance to learn, a brave and gracious patient was recruited from the GYN clinic.

It began with eight gloved students arranged in a semicircle behind the instructor who stood between the woman's legs doing his see-one, do-one routine. One at a time, we stepped in and went through the entire process while being critiqued by the instructor, all done as if the patient wasn't there at all.

When I finished, I said, "Thank you," to the patient, though her head was turned away, and she seemed not to notice. It is very different today. Now, student's first patient is a life-like manikin, no legs or torso, just a pelvis on a pedestal. After mastering manikins, students practice on paid "models," commonly used in teaching across specialties, before being allowed to touch "real" patients.

Obstetrics was divided between private and clinic patients. Our role with private patients was limited to sitting with patients in labor, and if invited by the patient, observing the birth itself. On the clinic side, we were slightly more involved, often delivering babies in routine cases, but mainly assigned to spend endless hours at night with patients in labor.

When a cesarean delivery was required, we held the retractors and watched. The first time I saw a C-section, I was stunned by the rapidity of the procedure. It was carefully orchestrated, starting the instant the anesthesiologist said the patient was unconscious. In about a minute, the surgeon exposed and opened the uterus, lifted the baby out, and handed the newborn to a nurse. The umbilical cord was cut, the baby handed over to the waiting pediatrician, and the surgeon then turned back to remove the placenta. In quick succession, bleeding vessels were tied, the uterus was stitched together, followed by closing the lining of the abdomen, the muscles that had been cut, and finally, the skin was closed—usually a job left for the intern or resident.

GYN surgery involved a lot of D&Cs, a relatively simple procedure to scrape the inside of a uterus, most often following a miscarriage. We were occasionally allowed to do some of the scraping part, something that took a careful touch to avoid damaging or even piercing the uterus. Abortions were done as well, often written off as "D&Cs." It was a touchy subject then as now, and some doctors, nurses, and anesthesiologists refused to have anything to do with it. Others were more pragmatic.

Two other OB-GYN observations, both related to sensitivity about intimacy. While not entirely taboo, conversations about a woman's sex life were still not considered part of a normal doctor-patient discussion. This was medical practice, not suitable for birds-and-bees sex talk. That attitude carried over directly into the way surgery was handled, especially when the surgery had profound effects on both the body and the patient's psyche. It was easy enough to tell a woman to refrain from intercourse for six weeks after surgery or childbirth, but beyond that, the focus was strictly clinical.

The most common major GYN procedure was the hysterectomy. For the surgeon, it was routine work. He (yes, he) saw the patient at the time of surgery and then some weeks later.

What was in-between wasn't discussed in any detail. Quite the opposite. Paucity of information about what was ahead conveyed the message, "There's nothing to it. Take it easy while you heal up. And look at the good part: no more periods." Such blandishments totally miss the effect sudden disruption has on a woman's endocrine system.

Because most hysterectomies leave at least one ovary, it was easy to be reassuring about long-term consequences. Two problems: even with the ovaries left in place, removal of the uterus is still a shock to the system and can produce a sudden array of menopausal symptoms. Also, ovaries and uterus have a common blood supply, and removing the uterus can starve the ovaries for blood, leading to hormonal disruption, and full-blown menopausal symptoms.

Breast cancer was always treated with surgery with or without radiation. The procedure was menacingly called, "Radical Mastectomy." Chemotherapy for breast cancer didn't really start to get off the ground until the 1970s. During my time in training, treatment was all about surgery. Talk about different types of limited surgery has only recently become part of the normal treatment picture, usually as part of a chemotherapy protocol. In the early 1960s, the standard was radical mastectomy: removal of the breast and lymph nodes, extending across the chest wall into the axilla—the arm pit. It was brutal, painful, and mutilating. What was missing was any discussion of the impact such a massive invasion had on the patient's mind as well as her body. To the extent it was talked about, surgery was presented as lifesaving. Wasn't that enough? Beyond that, you might want to talk to a psychiatrist. Most women were left to cope alone. Husbands were sympathetic, the same for friends, but anything below the surface, deeper in the woman's emotional world, was hers to cope with. Support groups were a novelty; stoicism and painful gratitude were the rule.

When I looked in our massive GYN textbook, I found only one paragraph in the entire book about anything vaguely concerned with a woman's feelings about sex. It said in condescending tone that occasionally a patient might ask the doctor a question about sexual matters. The author's advice was clear and to the point. In such cases the patient should be told to defer to her husband's preferences. Period. End of discussion.

After talking about this issue with a colleague, he called a retired gynecologist friend to ask if he had discussed sex after surgery with his patients. His answer: "I never asked."

After OB-GYN came surgery, a surprisingly different experience in both tone and pace. GYN procedures were usually planned, emergencies relatively infrequent, and OB seemed to be largely an exercise in waiting followed by a sudden burst of activity. Surgery was a different ball game, not just because of its rigorous schedule and blistering interrogations, but also because of the department's heavy-hitter faculty, each member seemingly with his own sense of drama. Warnings from a shrinking supply of upperclassmen were spot-on for once.

For starters, the department was seen as bigger than life by virtually everyone in the school, as well as the medical community beyond. It began on the first day we entered the main teaching hospital. There, at the main entrance, was an enormous portrait: the famous 1875 Thomas Eakins painting, *The Gross Clinic*, portraying famed Jefferson surgeon Samuel D. Gross Jr. performing surgery in the Jefferson surgical amphitheater. Gross is pictured holding a bloody scalpel over the patient while the poor man's mother cringes in the background. Rows of captivated students and physicians are arrayed in the steep bank of the theater behind Gross. Eakins painted himself into the portrait as a note-taking student. Like rubbing the Pieta's toe at the Vatican, it was said to be good luck for medical students to touch the frame as one walked by.[4]

The S.D. Gross incarnation in my time was Dr. John Gibbon, the first surgeon to perform open heart surgery using a machine

---

4. The 8' x 6.5' painting was sold to the Philadelphia Museum of Art in 2007 for $68,000,000, the money used for expansion of the medical school. A reproduction now hangs in place of the original.

allowing blood to continue to circulate while the heart was stopped for repair. Every year, Dr. Gibbon gave a lecture in the surgical pit complete with the original heart-lung machine, and Cecelia Bavolek, the first patient to undergo surgery with the complicated device. She was 18 at the time of the surgery in May 1953. She recovered nicely and lived another 30 years.

It was a magnificent moment. Drama, history, and a great outcome! All at *my* medical school! Maybe I was right to think this was the course to follow. It's funny how grandiosity can often push thoughtful reflection out of the way.

There were, of course, many lectures, but finally, the amazing moment standing elbow to elbow with surgeons. We scrubbed our fingers raw, walked into the operating room with hands held aloft to keep them from contamination, and when invited, took our place at the operating room table. One learned a lot in a hurry, starting with how to stand, belly against the table, hands up, all to enable one to maintain position without moving, maintaining enough leverage to hold and pull on retractors, literally for hours.

That was the good part. But this was a learning experience, and when not demanding instruments from the surgical nurse, or talking to the anesthesiologist about the patient's status, the surgeon grilled the residents, interns, and students, all standing in their specific place at the table. For routine work, the resident was in charge, but the drilling was the same, just the audience was smaller—and less embarrassing. It was harder work than I had realized, there was no joking or conversation at all, and everyone maintained total focus on the orchestrated performance.

As time went on, we were given a specific chore: cutting sutures for the surgeon. In even the most pedestrian operation there were dozens of suture knots tied, each one to be cut exactly to the length the surgeon wanted—or else. The surgeon would tie the knot, lift up the two pieces of suture together, and say, "Cut!" You didn't make a move until he said the magic word, then one moved with deliberate speed to cut the suture exactly the right distance from the knot.

"Too long."

"Too short."

One never seemed to get it right. Some surgeons were more tolerant than others, but cutting for the most demanding was like hearing, "Fool," or "Idiot," with every snip.

Once, one of my classmates, George Segal, experiencing several hours of "too long, too short," lost his senses, and failed to act when he was told to "Cut!" He just stood, unmoving, scissors just inches from the threads.

"I said, 'Cut!' What's the matter with you?"

"Well, sir," George said soberly, "I'm just trying to decide if I should make this one too long or too short."

He was thrown out on the spot, a hero to us, but seen in a less flattering way by the surgeons.

One of the most demanding of all was Dr. J.Y. Templeton, second-in-command to Dr. Gibbon; he took over the department when Dr. Gibbon retired in 1967. Dr. Templeton had a slightly southern accent and a sarcastic, sometimes caustic, teaching style. But watching him in the operating room was pure magic. His command of the room and all its players was absolute, and his manual dexterity—even to my completely inexperienced eyes—was stunning. Somehow, he could use both hands independently while maintaining continuous interaction with everyone at the table. He was a tough questioner, but there was always a slightly humorous edge to his banter. One of his famous quips, allegedly aimed at an intern, was that there was nothing in the human body he couldn't fix. Coming from any other surgeon, it would have been grandiose. From Templeton, it was less about what he could do than about what drove him, the motivation he wanted his students feel.

Like schools everywhere—graduate and otherwise—there were always a few students whose attention to learning was so intense, so total, the front seats in every lecture were theirs, the better to be seen with their hands in the air at every opportunity, seemingly indifferent to their sometimes abrasive, even discourteous, nature. Dr. Templeton never let them ruffle his feathers.

On one memorable day, he gave a lecture on surgical methods to stop bleeding in the esophagus, an extremely serious condition usually seen in patients with such severe liver disease the flow of blood into the liver is blocked. That produces "varices," engorged and fragile veins, like huge hemorrhoids, to bulge into the esophagus. If one ruptures, the patient can bleed to death in minutes. If the patient is lucky enough to be in a hospital at that moment, a slender, deflated balloon is inserted into the esophagus and inflated to temporarily stop the bleeding. But rapid surgery has to follow to tie off the bleeders. The subject that morning was about which was the best way to approach the veins: up from the abdomen or through the chest wall—either the "Trans-abdominal" or the "Trans-thoracic" route. Each side had its proponents. Dr. Templeton opined that he preferred the abdominal approach. He scarcely had the words out of his mouth when a hand shot up in the front row.

"Dr. Templeton! Sir!"

Like a buzzard looking down at a dead opossum, Dr. Templeton eyed the man, waited a few seconds, then said in his slow Virginia drawl, "Yes?"

"Sir. An article in the March issue of the *Journal of Thoracic Surgery* says that the *Harvard* Group" (heavy emphasis "Harvard") "prefers the trans-thoracic route of ligation of esophageal varices. Could you comment, Sir?"

Templeton allowed a slight smile to creep in, took another few seconds, leaned forward on the lectern, and said, "Well, young man, I simply wouldn't take my varices to that group."

Another one of his well-known moments—one I did not observe but heard about at the time—came during a gathering of the research committee, an annual meeting in which departments made their case for precious yearly funding allocations. One of the presenters was Dr. Sunderman, part of a father-son research team with a somewhat independent role based on their reputation for innovative research projects. The group, including Dr. Templeton, listened as Dr. Sunderman Sr. reviewed his proposal to study the heart function of the giraffe. His presentation was elegant, basically saying there was a lot to be learned from the power of the giraffe's heart.

"Witness the giraffe! His brain sits atop a six-hundred-pound, two-meter-long column of bone, muscle, sinew, nerves, and blood vessels. His twenty-five-pound heart is capable of pumping sixteen gallons of blood a minute up that neck to the brain. Imagine it!"

Dr. Templeton said he was indeed impressed, but asked, "Doctor Sundeman, did it ever occur to you that the giraffe might have his brain in his ass?"

I doubt anyone else could have gotten away with such a remark.[5]

Another event took place during my surgery rotation, though *at that point* it wasn't related to my studies (italics to indicate, *more to come*). It happened on my birthday. My wife planned a roast beef dinner, and I was going to take the evening off from study so we could better enjoy the moment. I was late getting out of the hospital, and as I came out onto the sidewalk ready to quick-step back to my house, I heard a voice—loud and clear.

"REPENT!!"

Dear God! I've heard that voice before. I turned and sure enough, there was John Jesus, Bible over his head, hectoring pedestrians about their sinful ways. I turned away, but it was too late.

"Brother Philip!" he yelled. I was busted right there on the sidewalk not fifty feet from Dr. Gross. Now it was my turn to cringe. He greeted me like a long-lost lamb, in an almost friendly way. He remembered my friend by name, and asked what I was doing. I said the obvious and quickly added that I was terribly late for dinner, hated to be rude, but I had to go. Next, my big mistake. He asked where I lived, said he might visit. I said "Camac Street," nothing more specific, and took off at a fast clip. He didn't follow.

---

5.   Dr. Templeton retired in 1987. A few years before his death in 2015, he underwent open heart surgery performed by one of his former students. He recovered and returned to his hobbies of hiking, fishing, and boatbuilding.

I got home, rushed upstairs to take a shower, eager to enjoy a relaxed evening. Suddenly my wife ripped open the shower curtain, her face purple with rage.

"Who the hell is John Jesus?!!" she demanded. "He's down in our living room preaching to me, yelling you told him where we live, and he's here to save us from sin!!"

I dressed in a hurry and went down to try to calm John who was full tilt in a fit of salvation excitement. I tried everything I could to get him out, and finally I literally pushed him out and locked the door. He did go away, but the meat was overcooked, and the evening was ruined. "At least," I thought, "that should be the end of it, and if I see him again in the street, I'll do what I can to avoid him." I didn't see John again, but that wasn't the end of our "relationship."

The third year morphed into the fourth, essentially a rerun of the tour of specialties, but this time with more hands-on experience. Internship was looming, we had to pass the second part of the National Boards, plus sharpen the skills we would need in the real, less-protected world of internship. The only diversion for me at school was a sidetrack job I undertook to work on our yearbook.

It probably sounds downright silly to imagine a yearbook in medical school; after all, that's what you expect in high school and college, not graduate school. But Jefferson had one, they needed help, and I was offered the job. It came with a $16K budget, and a guarantee the yearbook company would do 90% of the work. Just get some pictures, make up some clever captions, get a few faculty members to write something about our class, and you're done. We'd be grateful.

Oh, and one more thing: if you sell advertising and you take in more than you spend, you can keep the change for your trouble.

It struck me that because Jefferson had changed its policy to allow women to attend, starting the following fall, ours would be the last all-male class ever at Jefferson—or any other medical school in the country, for that matter. Four years later, Women's Medical College of Pennsylvania, also in Philadelphia, started to admit men. I gathered a few friends, and together we decided to see if we could capitalize on the effect—mostly negative—the change was having on alumni. Even better: we were told Jefferson had the largest number of living alumni of any US medical school. If it was even close to true, armed with names and addresses, and leaning on the nostalgia theme, we could potentially sell books well beyond the senior class.

We embellished the fact that Jefferson is the 10th oldest medical school in the country, stirred in plenty of sepia-colored 19th century photographs, padded the faculty essay section with several written by us under invented names, wrapped it in leather with gold lettering, and...Presto! *A unique book of memories, yours for only $15.*

The orders poured in, the money piled up, and in the end, our small staff split the considerable harvest.

With Part II of the National Boards out of the way, attention shifted to securing the right internship. True to form, I very nearly botched that one, too.

Because I was still under the influence of fantasy, I clung to the idea of becoming a surgeon, a plastic surgeon to be more exact. At that point I focused on two North Carolina internships linked to outstanding plastic surgery residencies. I visited both and came away with the understanding that if I listed them at the top of my order of preference list, I would stand a good chance of getting in. Instead of padding my list with the dozen or so I should have, I only added a third, also known for surgery, though its particular interest was in the emerging field of transplant surgery.

Looking back, I should have reckoned on the one factor that could trip me up: a less than stellar grade on the surgery section of the second National Board test at the end of senior year. I did well enough to get my third choice, bloody grateful to have it at all. Another irony: it's the same place where I had my disastrous electron microscope interview.

But I graduated, had a fine place to go, and while I had to eat crow about being ditched by the other two, in the end it turned out to be an incredibly good and equally undeserved piece of luck.

Like the story of George Segal cutting the surgeon's sutures, there is another such tale, one I heard about while interviewing at one of the plastic surgery programs. Had I looked past the humor, I might have seen the caution sign. Again, I missed it.

Part of the interview process meant attending morning "Pre-Op," a meeting of faculty, residents, and students to discuss the morning's scheduled surgery. The head of the department presided, his caustic remarks sparing no one. We had been pre-warned to remain invisible, allegedly because the chief was still fuming over a recent pre-op incident. True or not, the story was that the chief resident began by reading off the schedule, saying quickly that the first case was an inguinal hernia repair, the second case was…

"STOP," demanded the Chief. "Tell me, doctor: what exactly *is* a hernia?"

Asking the chief resident to explain a hernia is like asking Einstein what numbers are for. But the resident, obviously unperturbed by the intrusion, quickly answered.

"A hernia is the displacement of an organ or part of an organ from its normal area of confinement to an area outside of that area. Sir."

"Well, then," the Chief huffed, sticking out his tongue, "is this a hernia?"

"No, sir," the resident replied. "That's a hemorrhoid." As far-fetched as that sounds now, having witnessed a number of Pre-Op shows, the story probably is true.

Thank goodness for that one mediocre grade. Otherwise, I might have limped along hoping to outlast the misery and start a career. Who knows? But looking back, I'm happy that the sum of all mishaps, unforeseen twists, and lucky breaks did coalesce around a long and satisfying career.

Graduation was a dream come true, my parents were proud, and though I didn't know it at the time, it included one of those prescient twists of fate: the graduation speech was given by Anna Freud, daughter of Sigmund Freud.

But best of all, I received a congratulatory graduation card from Granny Cleek. She died six months later.

4

INTERNSHIP
CONFRONTING REALITY

THERE WAS PRECIOUS LITTLE TIME after graduation to savor the moment, move to a new city, and ready ourselves for the next step. While internship put all of us on the threshold of defining our career path, we first had to work through a new level of challenge, a dramatic shift from dealing in abstractions to the daunting realization that every answer could have an immediate impact on a patient's life. As we were told over and over: there was no time to look up an answer, and no room for error.

My work hours also meant a huge realignment of our family life, heaping more work on my wife, not only to maintain our home, do all of the shopping, cooking, childcare, and other day-to-day chores, but also to make sure my time off gave us a sense of living something approaching a normal family life. We had been spoiled by the relatively relaxed final year of school, and we both knew that was about to change.

We also had to turn in our lofty "Senior" status in medical school for a slot at the bottom of the physician hierarchy. I say "we" because my wife had been very much a part of everything I been through, and had herself become invested in school life outside of home, including serving as president of the now anachronistic Women's Auxiliary of the Student AMA. She and the other wives were keenly aware that tradition held internship to be relentless, pressured, a winnowing out of the unprepared now that the easy part—medical school—was out of the way. Command of the basics was assumed; the focus was now on how to apply that to the real world of diagnosis and treatment. All of it dictated studying on the nights I was home, especially in surgery where the morning's cases were daily quiz sessions. Our schedule was on-duty thirty-six hours, off-duty twelve, plus two weeks' vacation, all on a salary of $150 a month.

There have been many changes in the meaning and purpose of "Internship" in the years since its introduction after WWI. Before that, completing medical school was considered enough to allow licensing, provided one passed the necessary examinations. Passing Part III of the National Boards and completing internship still allows one to be licensed, but the idea of going directly into practice has disappeared. Getting malpractice insurance, hospital privileges, or being hired into an established practice would be impossible without residency training. The GP (General Practitioner) of old has faded away.

The word "internship" has also disappeared, replaced by "PGY-1," reflecting the idea that this is the first post graduate year of training, to be followed by PGY-2, PGY-3, and so on, depending on the residency. There has also been a change in the impact of the first year after medical school. "Internship" hosted a number of variations, concentrating on specific areas in preparation either to go directly into practice, or prepare for residency specialization. PGY-1 is more focused, reflecting the fact graduates today emerge with a clear idea of where they are headed, no need for the Whitman Sampler—go straight for the caramel.

There were, of course, many in our day who were already certain, and for them, there were "Straight" internships organized around a specialty. There were also "Mixed" and "Rotating" internships. "Mixed" was a step down from "Straight," focused on a specialty, but with other, complimenting areas mixed in. "Rotating" was just that: moving through the full gamut of disciplines. I chose the Rotating program, thrilled to be able to align the sequence of specialty departments to prepare for whatever was ahead. At that point, the surgery idea was starting to wilt, but I chose a two-month immersion at the start to settle the issue one way or the other. The rest was weighted on Internal Medicine—can't go wrong there—plus OB-GYN, pediatrics, and emergency work.

Before the intern-turned-practitioner faded out in the 1950s, there were an enormous number of GPs who went straightaway into practice, especially in rural areas where the doctor had to do just about everything from general medicine to obstetrical care, even emergency surgery. Without the GP, a huge number of smaller communities would have been underserved. Access to specialists was limited. When available at all, it was only because they rotated through medium-sized communities on a regular basis.

But how did the GPs of old do it? I asked that question in the mid-1950s to the GP who looked after the rural community in Virginia where Granny Cleek lived. She regaled me with stories about making her rounds in a horse-drawn buggy, delivering babies in barns and hayfields, setting bones, sewing up huge cuts, even doing some minor surgery. How did she do it? It was simple: "Back then, there just wasn't any choice."

Still, it had to be daunting. There must have been one thing that held it all together, some mantra that allowed her to be comfortable in such a risky setting. "You're right," she said. "The trick is: *you've got to know when to send 'em.*" You had to know what you didn't know and be prepared to act immediately. That was good old-fashioned wisdom then, and it still applies today.

From the late 18th to the middle of the 19th century, "medical school" was a pretty loose term. The basic teaching tool was an apprenticeship of about three years with an established physician. Admission to a school's didactic program was open to anyone with tuition money. In 1876, Johns Hopkins University increased its curriculum to four years, raised admission standards, and introduced the concept of "residency" for a select, elite group of postgraduate physicians. Other medical schools soon followed the Hopkins model.

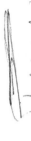

For many years, postgraduate training followed the hair-shirt model: long hours spent slaving away for either no salary or a pittance, undertaken in gratitude for the chance to learn, all aimed at starting a practice somewhere down the road. Usually, the loftier the status of the program, the less it paid. My subsistence salary was fairly typical for the time.

Major changes in hours worked and salary paid to medical staff changed dramatically starting in the late 1980s, largely the consequence of a well-publicized medical catastrophe.

An 18-year-old college student, Libby Zion, was admitted to a New York City hospital in a state of collapse, disoriented, and dehydrated. She deteriorated and died, though the exact cause of her death was not immediately clear. Her father was a prominent lawyer who—along with many others—felt her care had been negligent, largely a consequence of being in the hands of exhausted residents. A protracted investigation and lawsuit followed, and as a consequence of both, a series of rules for interns and residents was enacted in 1989. The standards dictated no more than 80 hours of work a week, a maximum of 24 hours straight duty, 1 day off a week, and no more than one night duty every three days. Because interns were seen as having such heavy workloads, in 2003 their shifts were limited to 16 hours.

It sounded good, but the system had its drawbacks, starting with truncated care. Instead of a physician being able to stay with a patient for a longer stretch, the patient had to be handed off to someone else at the end of each shift. It also had a significant effect on physician education. Studies in 2003 muddied the issue further by failing to show any specific set of changes improved either patient care or staff education. Debate, study, and experimentation followed, adding complexity without real benefit. Some of the sillier ideas were: requiring physicians to leave the facility after each shift, plus mandated courses in "Alertness Management" and "Strategic Napping." In 2017, the 16-hour limit was lifted to allow interns a full 24 hours per shift. The 80-hour week with one day off was kept, along with the limit of one night every three days.

In a parallel movement, interns and residents rebelled against poverty wages, demanding and finally receiving better pay. Currently, the average pay is around $50,000 a year, not at all unreasonable when you factor in the cost of living coupled with the near universal need to service accumulated debt.

For us, debt was not the issue it is today, the cost of living was dramatically lower, and we counted ourselves fortunate to be able learn from great teachers in highly academic settings. Today, it is hard to find and compensate experienced clinicians who delight in teaching. Institutions struggle for money, in large measure because the cost of hospital care is barely covered by myriad insurance and government-supervised income streams. No insurance source will compensate medical staff not directly involved in a specific patient's care. Also, in today's world, residents spend hardly any time with patients, much less in learning situations not related to procedures. No matter how gifted teachers may be, they all have their own struggles with the universal parsimony of today's scattered system.

Rebellion was the last thing on our minds in 1964. We accepted the lousy pay and did not object to being on duty 36 hours and off 12 hours. It was just part of the deal. We all did it. And being on 36 hours did not mean we got zero sleep in that time. In fact, we all had basic but comfortable rooms in the staff dormitory, the place where we also took our meals. We slept between events, and helped each other out if one member of the group had been up all night. It was a system of taking care of each other as well as our patients.

Within each small group, we took patients in rotation, but did rounds together twice a day, constantly talking about all of the patients under our immediate care, and routinely filling in for each other when needed. Though paperwork was confined to the patient's chart, there was nothing casual about that system. Proper documentation was an absolute necessity, guided by one overarching principle: notes were adequate only when they were *legible* and so *complete* that a new physician, one absolutely ignorant of a patient's status, could read the chart and *seamlessly continue care.*

Today, the computer rules, and the end of each shift is taken up with recording everything in the computer. About 40% of each shift is spent on the computer. The same dean who told me that fact added, "Next time you are in a hospital walking by the nurses' station, notice just how many of the medical staff are fastened to a computer screen." Those same computers are loaded with algorithms, too. Physicians feed in the data and the computer suggests what to do next. It is easy to see other advantages of the new system: computers remember the potential side effects of all drugs, don't get tired, forget something, or miss a zebra diagnosis.

Another difference, one that can be seen either as a plus or a minus, is interns don't get distracted by bedside chores like drawing blood, starting an IV, or doing a spinal tap. They may have drawn blood a few times in medical school, but they haven't done it over and over to the point of being able to hit a tiny vessel in a severely dehydrated heroin addict in acute withdrawal—the gold standard of tough draws. And they absolutely do not go for the femoral vein, even when other veins are out of play.[1]

"So what?" you might ask. The new way is more efficient, frees the intern to finish paperwork, and the learning part is still intense and ultimately focused on providing good care. Totally true, though the old system did mean more time interacting with our patients and their family; hard to quantify, but essential to building trust. Doing procedures, or "scut work" as it was called, was simply part of the process.

---

1.   The femoral is the large vein coming out of the leg at the groin, sitting just inside the femoral artery and the femoral nerve. The sequence is nerve-artery-vein, so if one feels the pulsing artery just below the junction of leg and abdomen, presses down between the artery and vein to protect the artery, a needle can safely be inserted into the vein. Blood flows easily from the large vein, and the artery is in no danger. We did it fairly routinely; today, it is rarely done.

None of us talked about future practice in terms of money. I think it's fair to say we simply assumed that finding our place in the profession would take care of itself. In fairness to today's trainee's focus on money, it should be pointed out that we did have one advantage. In the 1950s and 1960s, deserving college students got scholarships, and medical school was amazingly inexpensive. So while it was a tough financial slog through post graduate training, at least it wasn't also burdened with enormous accumulated debt.

My internship was at the Medical College of Virginia in Richmond. Looking around at the interns gathered on that first day, I saw a familiar group; again, all male and all white, a continuation of college and medical school. It is shocking not only to realize that African Americans were essentially iced out of both then, but a half a century later, they still only represent 7.7% of all medical students.

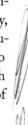

Women have done a lot better. In 1960, the number of women enrollees was 7%. By 1982, it had risen to 27%. Today, by a 1% margin, there are more women entering medical school than men. Fifty years ago, female faculty members were a rarity; today, the number is nearly 40%.

The exact current distribution among ethnic groups is surprisingly difficult to pin down. That said, Whites represent between 52% and 57%; Asians, between 22% and 25%; African Americans, 7–8%; Latinos, 6–9%; Native Americans, around 0.3%. Even through the surprising variation between sources, it is clear Whites and Asians dominate, while Latino and African American representation in only slowly improving.

White dominance is eroding, largely because of a surge in Asian applications. As a group, Asian students are highly motivated, have high grades, science majors, and approach the MCAT entrance exam with a laser-like focus. African Americans and Latin Americans do not do as well on the test; not surprising, when you think about the socio-economic and cultural hurdles they must clear just to get the opportunity to take the exam. However, when African American and Latin Americans are admitted to medical school with lower scores, they quickly become the academic equal of all of the other students, results born out in graduation rates. Entrance standards may have some flex, but graduation standards do not.

It's stunning to look back now and realize how totally unaware we were of issues like race, gender, and working conditions. Our all-male, all-white focus was only on what was just ahead. For me, there was growing apprehension over the fantasy of becoming a surgeon. I simply didn't have anything approaching Templeton's dedication, to say nothing of my frankly less-than-stellar performance on the surgery section of the National Boards. I felt like I was back in the morgue line talking to the fellow from Thiel College on the first day of medical school. He knew exactly where he was going—and I was clueless.

Same deal all over again, and the more I heard about the surgery program and its Chief, Dr. David Hume, the more my knees shook. Hume was a driven researcher, unflinchingly confident, a figure like Drs. Gibbon and Templeton, men who set the tone for everything and everyone in their department.

Hume performed the first successful kidney transplant in 1957, but his interests seemed to go everywhere from obscure endocrine disorders to heart transplants. The school historian confirmed my memory of Hume as an abrasive tyrant who drove his residents relentlessly. The hospital is within walking distance of the governor's house; convenient, because when Hume wanted something, he went straightaway to see the Head Man, made his demand—and always got what he was after. His Members Only group of interns, residents, and fellows were all infused with Hume's variation of drive. I had chosen to do my surgery rotation first, so I was about to find out if I had been a foolish dreamer, or just needed a good push to stop wondering and start working.

Before plunging into our rotations, we worked through an extensive orientation program, a series of lectures over several days, starting with senior staff introductions (minus Dr. Hume) and general rules, all with heavy emphasis on personal and professional responsibility. We began to learn our way around the 36 square blocks encasing the complex of several hospitals, medical school, library, laboratories, and related buildings, most of it connected by a tangle of underground passages.

Then attention turned to patient care, from general principles to the finest detail of how to calculate the electrolytes needed to individualize IV solutions. Happily, newer, prepared IV solutions with names like Ringer's Lactate were available, and the need to premix IVs was fading out—a real time saver. We learned the precise standards of care for specific common problems like heart attack, stroke, seizure disorders, and diabetes, plus guidelines for ordering lab work, and more—all the way down to the very last item on the list: handling the death of a patient.

You might think that last lecture would have come from the chaplain, but it came from a pathologist. The reason had nothing to do with dealing with distraught relatives, notifications, documentation, or even how to fill out a death certificate. No, it was focused on the autopsy expected when a patient died.

While the postmortem of one's patient was wrenching, it was the ultimate teaching device. You took care of the patient, did your best to restore health, but he had died, so your next step was participating in the autopsy to learn as much as possible about his illness, and the ultimate cause of death. Teaching hospitals were rated in part on the percentage of autopsies done. Other factors being equal, potential pathology residents were likely to bypass programs with a mediocre autopsy score.

There was just one little catch: you had to get the family's permission for the postmortem examination, and that wasn't always easy. Keeping the family informed about a patient's progress was a key part of developing trust; it also played a role in getting permission for autopsy. There were no HIPPA restrictions to stiffen interaction with the family. It was the opposite: keeping the family informed was part of providing good patient care. No one whined about it being unseemly or taking too much time; on the contrary, information gathered from family members was an integral part of clinical notes.

Over time, but still ahead of HIPPA, talking to families gave way to caution about medical-legal issues, another way of saying "malpractice." Caution gradually morphed into rationalizations to prevent it altogether. Enter "ethicists," experts who preached that what we saw as common sense was anything but. Documentation became statements laced with cautious phrasing, elevating malpractice prevention to a level equal to medical accuracy. There was pressure applied through malpractice attorneys to beef up documentation to suit their needs, specific references needed to thwart the threat of a lawsuit.

The lawyer who told us he could make Mother Teresa look like an ax murderer also told us the new gold standard for proper documentation: "Always write your notes expecting you will hear them again when they're read to a jury." And if they're helpful for the patient, that's good, too.

As that system strengthened, so did the role of didactic ethics, taught by a group of well-paid consultants. There was an exact parallel between the growth of HIPPA thinking and its progenitors: medical lawyers and ethicists. It began slowly with a few lectures, pretty obvious stuff, but like a kid's lava science project gone wrong, it increased exponentially, its arcane riddles becoming more convoluted and less intuitive. You couldn't sell the obvious; no one pays $300 for a day for that. No, the hook was to present a series of hypothetical dilemmas whose solution could only be divined by the presenter.

Ethics did have a problem, however: it was supposed to be a lofty, immutable guide approaching the durability of the Ten Commandments. But ethics needed a way to keep up with rule changes, not the other way around. So, what was ethical five years ago could be unethical today, seemingly without contradiction. Medical Ethics became the stalking horse of political correctness, purposely made obscure to convey gravitas, disguise its changeable nature, and reinforce the need for a cadre of experts to both translate for the gullible, and satisfy bureaucratic requirements.

As the ethics movement roared along, it became mandatory, part of every aspect of training as well as a yearly test requirement in institutions and continuing medical education programs. It consumed increasing time and precious resources, until it broke the system. The professionals disappeared, their tests jumped into computers, and the entire enterprise became just another nuisance, another meal for an already bloated cryptocracy.

It's a darn good thing we didn't have the Ethics Police watching us plead our case for autopsies. While we were usually able to get permission, there were times a family dug in and simply wouldn't budge.

Time to call Gomez.

Gomez was an Internal Medicine resident, a handsome Columbian man with a slight Latin accent, and an outsized charm gene. He was our go-to guy when all else failed, his technique a thing of incredible beauty. He would sweep into the room, go from relative to relative, never missing the smallest child, each receiving his most sincere sympathy over their loss. He would then encourage some talk about the deceased, quoting compliments and other flatteries to make it clear the deceased was a special person to all of us. He never used the toxic word "autopsy," offering instead "postmortem" in a way that suggested it was not much more than another physical examination. He said nothing about the reality of taking the patient apart on a cold steel table. Even when the postmortem was rejected, Gomez seemed undaunted; in fact, he would appear to embrace the family's decision, saying he understood exactly how they felt.

If the family was sophisticated and well informed, Gomez had a specific line of persuasion. Here, the appeal was to what the patient would have wanted. After all, he valued education above all, and the idea he could—even in death—make a contribution to medical education, well, he certainly would have embraced it, don't you think?

Most of our patients were, however, far from well off. Ours was largely a charity operation, and our patients were generally poor, not well educated, and in those moments, distraught. All of it came together in Gomez's next move.

It began slowly. He would stand up, smile, and say again how badly he felt, assuring the family the body could soon be released to the undertaker. Then he made his Colombo move: "Oh," he would say with a quick slap to his forehead, a sudden afterthought as he headed for the door. "Chu can haf de body, but you know he had a berry, berry bad impection, so you got to bury him in de ocean." He would explain that such an infection could easily spread to mourners, too great a risk to take. But there was one alternative: if the family agreed to the autopsy, we would be able to remove the infection, and they could bury him properly—and safely.

While I didn't see it, it was said he had an alternative ploy for patients who had received radiation treatment. In that one, the family was told the radiation concentrated in the brain, so they could have the body, but not the head, unless, of course, they signed, and let us decontaminate the head.

Gomez never missed, and I am not aware of anyone ever complaining about his methods.

The death of a patient offered other learning opportunities. As soon as the patient died, the curtain was drawn around the bed so we could practice procedures, initially under the guidance of a resident; later, on our own. We did intubations (opening the breathing passage to insert a tube), tracheotomies, femoral stabs (to draw blood from the groin area), spinal taps, cut-downs (finding a vein by opening the skin), and boldest of all: the liver biopsy. That memory is so vivid I even remember the names of the biopsy needles we used: Vim Silverman and Manghini. I was startled to learn they are both still used today.

During those first days, we were reminded of another elephant in the waiting room, one I hadn't seriously considered before: the draft. It was suddenly clear we needed to know our options, and make some decisions in the next several months. The Vietnam War was raging, and all physicians were subject to being drafted into the Army for two years at the end of internship. The only way around it was the Berry Plan, a deferment based on already being in or accepted in a residency program. Deferments allowed three years to complete training before being drafted. But there was a snag: to make up for the deferment break, you owed three years to the Army, not the two years required following internship. Like many of my colleagues, I didn't qualify for the Berry Plan, and it was unlikely I would figure out my specialty path and get a residency commitment in six months—the time before draft notices would arrive.

Being armed with solid experience in basic disciplines, I reasoned, would prepare me for whatever the Army had in store. There was also another option: the Public Health Service (PHS). While accepting a commission in the PHS avoided the draft and the near certainty of being sent to a war zone, it was also a long-term commitment, a career choice offering the satisfaction of providing health care to an underserved population here in the USA. Also, with acceptance in the PHS, I might be able to leverage a good assignment in the Army, trade up, and keep my option open for a new specialty path.

There was one other curve ball to deal with, another pitch I somehow hadn't seen coming, or had foolishly minimized. In our tours of the various specialty areas, it suddenly dawned on me that our institution was still thoroughly segregated.

This was July 1964. *Brown vs. Board of Education* had been decided unanimously by the Supreme Court ten years before. One day after I arrived in the program, President Johnson signed the Civil Rights Act, and three months later, Martin Luther King Jr. won the Nobel Peace Prize. I had come from the North, where there were only tinges of overt racism showing, to a large southern city, capital of the state, where the Civil War was referred to as, "The War of Northern Aggression," and a popular bumper sticker read: "A good Yankee is like a hemorrhoid that comes down and then retreats." I simply wasn't aware or remotely ready for it. Interestingly, exactly one month after I completed the program in June 1965, the hospital dropped every vestige of segregation. But being confronted with the full-on force of segregation in the first moments of the program made me feel like I was living another anachronism, like being in the last all-male class in an American medical school. But there it was, and I had to deal with it.

There was no segregation in Philadelphia, but there were plenty of subtle forms of prejudice, just not the 12-gauge, government supported onslaught I suddenly met just a few states away. Like most cities, Philly was divided into distinct ethnic neighborhoods, reflecting three hundred years of evolution, ethnic grouping, mercantile pressures, and more. The strongest and most geographically defined were Italian and African American neighborhoods. Jefferson was close to the edge of both, and our house was only a half block from Lombard Street, one block before South Street, the understood borderline of the Black neighborhood, an area one didn't venture into alone at night. Crime was rampant, but less troublesome in our immediate area than it was a few blocks south. Still, there was the night a woman was stabbed to death at the end of our block, right near the line. Who knows why?

Crime, incidentally, came in two forms: random and mob related. Historically, Philadelphia was a pretty corrupt place. Even in the early 1960s, there were mob-run speakeasy establishments meant to circumnavigate Philadelphia's antiquated Blue Laws, especially rules for alcohol use. No booze was sold from midnight on Saturday until Monday morning. Night life was either in hidden "clubs" or over the bridge in Cherry Hill, New Jersey.

Some city officials, especially in the police ranks, hardly bothered to disguise their greed. One evening my wife and I decided to have a beer at Franks, our neighborhood bar, a small, unadorned place dominated by a horseshoe-shaped bar, a few tables and chairs—but nothing else. We were about to leave when three cops suddenly appeared. Two covered the doors and one confronted Frank at the bar. No one would be allowed to leave until Frank paid fifty dollars.

"What!" Frank protested. "I just paid you three days ago!"

Too bad, he was told. Fifty bucks to open the doors. Frank didn't have fifty in the till, so his customers took up a collection. The cops took their money, and we went home to eat.

Frank's was also an all-white bar, not because of overt discrimination, but because of a kind of unspoken understanding. Just two blocks away on the edge of the African American section, there was another bar, the Rainbow, and it was all Black. Same understanding. But they had entertainment, local musicians who randomly turned up to play. A kid circulated around selling fried chicken: one piece of chicken between two pieces of white bread for fifty cents. The reason I know is because I was invited to go there one night with a man who worked in the hospital. No one seemed to notice me or care, and the music was great—so was the chicken.

In our neighborhood, medical students and anyone else wearing a white jacket with a stethoscope in one pocket, was not in any danger. The reason was simple: Jefferson served all citizens in the surrounding area without any concern for race or ability to pay. Everyone understood it, and in my four years, I never heard of a single assault on any member of the medical community.

There was more overt racism among some members of my family than I saw in my entire Philadelphia experience, though none of it prepared me for life in a totally segregated institution. Most of the interns and a considerable proportion of residents in the program came from southern backgrounds and schools. They had seen and achieved some level of comfort with the system in the South. No one asked me if I had any apprehension about working in a segregated setting. Either it wasn't important enough to mention, or it was assumed I knew and didn't care.

I quickly learned to keep my mouth shut, focus on the work, and save my comments for selected conversations with fellow Yankees.

My next jolt was realizing there were two widely separated emergency departments, one for whites only, and the other for everyone else. Caught in the middle were Native Americans, members of several tribes with population centers near our institution. By state law, they were seen as Black, but when it came to which emergency room they were sent to, the decision was usually made by police and ambulance drivers. The ultimate filter, however, was in the hands of the clerks who registered incoming patients. If a Native American was brought to the white ER, and the on-duty clerk objected, the patient was sent around the block to the Black ER. The two-ER system dictated two month's training: one in each ER.

The ERs themselves were completely different worlds. The white ER was considerably smaller, quieter, and there were even times when there were no patients there at all, time to read, talk, and drink coffee. The Black ER was in another universe, much larger, always busy day and night. The reason had less to do with emergencies than about discrimination in medical care. There was no Medicaid in effect at that point, and the miniscule amount of health insurance available was well beyond the grasp of anyone in the enormous, impoverished population of the city. That meant the ER was the only option for health care, urgent or not. Medical care was relatively cheap, and a teaching hospital also meant little pressure was exerted to collect overdue bills. Medicare rules later made debt forgiveness a crime, forcing hospitals to aggressively pursue patients. Coupled with the absurd cost of care, ER treatment is today a major cause of financial catastrophe.

In stark contrast, white people generally had better access to outpatient services, were less inclined to use the ER for primary care, and could better handle fees. In the white ER, one could go an entire shift dealing with asthma attacks and sewing up cuts without consulting or even seeing a resident. On the other side of the hospital, residents—even faculty—were a constant feature.

At times, when there was an accident forcing emergency surgery right on the spot, and survival was in doubt, there was a strong likelihood surgical residents would show up with iced organ containers, anticipating a possible organ "donation" for research purposes, or perhaps match a kidney with one of several potential recipients, some actually living close by in hopes of receiving a life-saving match.

Putting quotes around "donation" is necessary because the system of gathering organs was still in its incipience. People making the decision to donate ahead of an untimely death were a rarity. Permission, when it was obtained at all, was often just verbal, there being little chance the person giving consent had the foggiest idea what was being asked, or was in any shape to think it through. It was presented as part of the emergency, and a strong likelihood the harvest was already under way.

One night, as residents were trying to save a man with grievous injuries from a car accident, a resident showed up with a cooler, leaned over to look at the patient, and said matter-of-factly to the residents working on the man, "Gone, don't you think?" The meaning was both clear and chilling. Indeed, shortly after that, the man was pronounced dead, interns and nurses left the room, and I presume an organ was taken, perhaps after getting something approaching permission.

I don't know how that one turned out, but in researching the issue, the hospital historian confirmed harvesting did indeed happen, and was both known and tolerated. Transplants were new, and above all else, they offered hope, especially for the multitude of kidney failure patients hanging on, living in the coalescing stricture of endless rounds of dialysis treatment. Such pioneering programs attracted skillful, daring, and innovative surgeons, plus an enormous surge of research money.

Changes in the rules and ethics had hardly kept up with the enthusiasm and momentum of the new game. It's no surprise the sketchy harvesting practice was not only tolerated, but within the inner circle of transplant physicians, quietly understood to be necessary.

You might reason that if organs had been taken, the undertakers might blow the whistle, say something—make a stink. Not so,

I was to find out. Theirs was a business, and they wasted no time matching the patient's surgical wounds with the cause of death. I never saw anything approaching that in the white ER. Remember, too, that families almost never have an idea about undertakers ahead of a fatal event. A lot of business came as referrals from our staff. Morticians didn't want to mess up a good system with unnecessary complaints.

There were two other distinctions between the two emergency worlds, starting with the "strong room" in the Black ER. "Strong room" was a euphemism for "jail cell," a place for patients deemed too unruly to be treated until they calmed down, sobered up, or were hauled away by the police. There was no jail cell in the white ER.

The other major difference was a six-bed "PID room" for female patients suffering from acute Pelvic Inflammatory Disease; in other words, a raging case of gonorrhea. PID was rampant, and while treatable with antibiotics, in its acute form it was excruciatingly painful, often accompanied by high fever and disorientation. Worse, untreated, secondary infection could quickly spread to the eyes and joints. In short, it was a true emergency requiring IV medication, fluids, and pain control.

The fact there was no PID room in the white end of the system confirmed the reasonableness of a racial bias in the minds of those unwilling to confront other realities. Plenty of white patients got gonorrhea, too, but they had better access to health care in the private sector, thus more likely to be treated early in the game before their STD advanced to the critical stage. Also, there was geographic selection: our hospital was a public institution in a poorer part of the inner city. White patients were more likely to live in areas served by more exclusive hospitals where discretion was part of the bargain.

There had been two nursing schools, one Black, the other white, until 1957 when they began to integrate. The key word is "began." The process wasn't complete until 1962. Initially, Black students were allowed but not welcomed in the white nursing school, and whites did not attend the Black school at all. That system finally imploded when a Black student became the class valedictorian in the predominantly white school. The class graduation party was held in a restaurant, but the valedictorian was not allowed to enter. She would have none of it, and in the ensuing uproar, the two-school, two-class system was finally buried.

Sadly, that did not end the bias against Black nurses. They were not welcome in local eateries or on predominantly white hospital wards. When I arrived, a sort of residual segregation remained, with Black patients in one place with Black nurses, and the rest, lily white. Incidentally, the OB service was integrated, apparently ahead of the curve. How progressive, I thought at the time. Not so, my research revealed. Two years before, the Black OB hospital section was forced to close because of rat infestation.

With orientation under our belts, we spread out to begin work. I was sent to the surgery floor, thinking there might be something of a welcome, maybe a chance to meet Dr. Hume, hear about the program. Not so. I walked onto the appointed ward, met the resident I was to shadow, and that was it. Rather than being grilled or lectured, I joined the train of residents and nurses just ahead of the caboose. The last car was always reserved for medical students.

My time in the surgery rotation, with one exception, turned out to be hugely helpful in teaching me the fundamentals of surgical practice. Because the residents assigned to intern duty were all just out of internship themselves, they had a certain sympathy for our situation. They pushed, but they didn't badger us, making it possible to let go of the anxiety and focus on the work.

This was truly the land of "Do One." Because of their junior status, new residents were given the simplest, most repetitive operative tasks. Lancing boils, treating wound infection, coping with burns, suturing more complex wounds, doing appendectomies, hernia repair, sigmoidoscopy, and hemorrhoid surgery took up most of our time. We were also frequently called to ERs to evaluate cases, an invaluable asset in learning the basics of emergency care. I was fortunate to have that experience first, well ahead of being assigned to an ER with no mentor at my side.

My first really big shock came about three weeks into the rotation. The resident was assigned to do several simple surgeries in a row, starting with a hemorrhoidectomy. I had seen and done the procedure a number of times with the resident, but this time I was told to do it myself while he watched. A few minutes in, he said he thought I could handle it, and left the OR. There I was, sitting on a stool, a nurse next to me, anesthesiologist lost somewhere in the sheets at the man's head, and the resident off on another case. It was another "Holy shit!" moment, but there was nothing to be done about it but continue. When I finished and the patient was taken away, I couldn't help thinking about the guy whose foot I had stitched together in medical school. Was I responsible for one man who couldn't walk straight, and another who would never have another normal Sunday morning with the *Times-Dispatch?* I took care of him while he recovered, and happily, he survived with a back door that still opened and closed normally.

In spite of all the positive learning, I did realize as I went along that I definitely was not cut out to be a surgeon. As much as I appreciated and enjoyed the process, I knew I was light years away from being drawn to the rigors of high voltage surgery, and the reality of repetition stretched out over the years ahead in a more typical general surgery practice told me it was time to move along.

Just a few days before the end of the rotation, I was mysteriously paired solo on a complex radical neck dissection with Dr. Hume's right-hand senior resident, Richard Cleveland, reputedly one of only a few who could get away with disagreeing with the Chief. It was a terrible three hours. He grilled and humiliated me from start to finish. I did my best, but there was no escaping the fact I was way out of my depth. At the end, he said he was glad to know I didn't have plans to try to be a surgeon. I told him I was just as glad as he was.

Dr. Cleveland went on to distinguished career, eventually becoming Chief of Surgery at Tufts-New England Medical Center.

He died of a brain tumor in 2002. A colleague described Dr. Cleveland as a brilliant surgeon, "at times gruff, and always a presence."

Dr. Hume died in 1972 when the single engine plane he was piloting crashed in the Santa Susana Mountains near Van Nuys, California. The weather was terrible, Hume did not have an instrument rating, and he dismissed advice to wait until the weather cleared. He was 55 years old.

The transition to Internal Medicine was dramatic. The focus went from procedures to diagnosis, from teaching by mentor to group discussion, and treatment was suddenly dependent on a huge number of possible medications and combinations, each with its own benefits and perils. In surgery, the anesthesiologist handled most of the dicey medications, and drug interactions were not a constant menace. Serious infection, heart disease, severe diabetes, and endocrine disorders all brought Internal Medicine specialists into play.

Each medical ward had its own chief, usually a senior member of the faculty. Medical residents, interns, and medical students made up the rest of the team. The atmosphere was collegial, and cases were distributed to give each of us experience with all types of illness. The situation today is quite different. The team structure is theoretically the same, but computers and insurance have altered the pace and, with it, teaching time at every level.

In today's world, the computer rules, stealing time away from patient interaction, isolating one staff member from another, and severely limiting the opportunity for group discussion. Behind it all is the constant pressure to get patients out of the hospital. Even in non-teaching hospitals where patients are taken care of by "hospitalists," the same pressure exists to live on a computer screen and get patients out before the QA monitors come nosing around demanding to know why Mr. Jones hasn't been discharged.

The hospitalist innovation, like every other device organized to solve a problem, has its own unintended issues. In the not-so-remote past, the doctor who took care of you in the office was the one who saw you through your hospital stay. Doctors rotated night duty within their practice, so even if the admitting physician was not your own, it was someone you knew, a partner with easy access to your regular physician who would take over your case in the morning. Today, the hospitalist starts from scratch, and the patient—already quite miserable—suddenly has to add uncertainty about the physician to his worries.

We were fortunate in having time to see patients through the entire treatment process, do repetitive examinations, study laboratory results, and most importantly: consult with team members as a matter of course.

My time in Internal Medicine included outpatient clinic work, sometimes seeing patients we had cared for on the inpatient ward. While under the Internal Medicine umbrella, I was also exposed to cardiology, some radiology, even a smattering of dermatology. Later, I would have a solid month on neurology. None of that would be hugely different in a PGY-1 Internal Medicine, Family Practice, or Primary Care residency today where diverse experience is still the rule.

Fellow interns quickly became friends and, married or not, formed the basis of our social life outside the hospital. We shared stories about experience across specialty areas, talked about the residents and faculty one could trust—or fear—and routinely covered for each other. One friend, Alan Cohen, a Straight Medicine intern, had taken a psychiatry rotation in August (important part of the story) as part of his program. Alan was endlessly cheerful, funny, and quick witted, as the following story will illustrate.

The inpatient psychiatry unit had a strong room similar to the one in the Black ER. One day, a large, angry, floridly psychotic truck driver was brought to the emergency room by police, but because he was so out of control, he was taken directly to the psychiatric unit to be placed in the strong room until they could figure out how to load him up with Thorazine. It took two cops and several attendants to get him to the floor, but when he saw the cell they were trying to push him into, he fought back even harder.

Alan stepped between the man and the open door, and said reassuringly, "See? It's perfectly safe in there, nothing to fear!" With that, the man lunged forward, pushed Alan into the cell, slammed the door behind him, pulled out a knife, and said, "I'm gunna cut your f...g throat."

Without missing a beat, Alan said, "You can't, it's snowing."

The man stopped, his already derailed thinking momentarily thrown off by Alan's bizarre statement. An attendant got the door open, the man was subdued, and Alan was freed. When I asked Alan why he said what he did, he shrugged and confessed he had no idea where it came from. In fact, one of the hallmarks of psychosis, particularly in schizophrenia, is a problem with *association*, the sequencing of thoughts in a logical progression. When something jars that system, it can instantaneously disrupt intention mid-thought. Had Alan said something soothing that didn't penetrate, he almost certainly would have been injured or killed.

I can't leave Alan without telling one more story, even though it is only tangentially related to training. We lived in the west end of town just a few blocks away from Alan. The quiet street was called a "parkway" because it was divided by a wide island of grass and shrubs. We had another neighbor, one I did not know, a friend of Alan's from high school, a fellow with a strange hobby. He collected snakes, not the baby boa variety, but venomous serpents, including cobras, and the worst of the bunch: a Blue Krait, one of the most venomous snakes in the world. He kept his collection in his basement, all carefully caged. There was one window, usually left ajar for ventilation.

One morning, he went to check on his pals and found a cobra missing from its cage. Apparently, the lid wasn't properly latched, and the snake pushed it open enough to slither through. He quickly—and carefully—searched the basement but didn't find the creature. He realized at that point the snake had slipped out the window and was loose in the neighborhood. In his panic, he called his level-headed friend, Alan. What should he do??!!! Look for the snake, hoping he could find it and somehow catch or kill it? Call the police and set off a neighborhood panic, plus get himself in trouble for owning several illegal snakes? And what if it bites someone?!

Alan said he *had* to call the cops, and in the meantime, yes, start looking. And, no, Alan was not inclined to help. I told you he was level-headed. The man decided to search first, give it an hour, and if that failed, he would have to call the police. He looked all around his house, yard, and garage, gradually expanding his search to the street. There were deep ditches on both sides, shaded and wet, ideal for snakes. Down the parkway, he saw a city worker walking in the ditch, cutting weeds with a sickle. He ran down and asked the man if he had seen any snakes in the last hour or so?

"Snakes? Are you kidding? I see snakes all the time. Fact is, I seen one a while ago. Son-of-a-bitch jumped up in front of me and started hissing. I said, 'No freaking snake hisses at me'," and making a sweeping motion with his sickle, said, "So I cut his f...g head off."

Sure enough, the decapitated cobra was right where the man said it was. It gave me a jolt when Alan told me the tale, just thinking the thing could have slithered its way just one more block to our house.

There was another intern in our small group who achieved a different kind of fame, a stunt that nearly got him thrown out. Go to acting school and leave medicine alone.

While most of our work was on the teaching wards, well away from private patients in the main hospital, occasionally a resident was called by a private physician to do something for a patient. Only when a resident couldn't respond would one of us be dispatched. It was a distraction none of us—resident or intern—wanted.

One afternoon, a fellow intern, David, was called to give a patient an injection to ease a breathing problem. It required a serious hike to the main hospital, up to the floor, then time to study the chart enough to know what was required. When David arrived, he was greeted by a nursing instructor leading a group of four nursing students in starched white attire, their very first day of nursing school. Since the patient was unconscious, it was felt that watching the injection would be a quiet, non-threatening way to get started.

David's irritation gave way to his sense of drama, and he rather grandly asked the students to arrange themselves at the foot of the bed. He began by telling them he would be giving the 88-year-old moribund patient an intravenous injection of aminophylline, explaining the potent drug is used to dilate small, constricted parts of the lung's breathing tubules. It must be given slowly or there is a risk of seizures or even sudden death from cardiac or pulmonary complications, especially in debilitated patients like this one. Pause to let "sudden death" sink in. Then as the students watched, he held the bottle of medication aloft, inserted the needle, and slowly filled the syringe. Turning to the patient, he snapped a tourniquet in place, found small vein, and wiped the skin with an alcohol sponge. He tapped the barrel to get the air bubble to rise, then carefully pressed the plunder, forcing out the air, plus a little squirt of the drug just for effect. The students cringed as he inserted the needle, pulled back the plunger to see a little blood, unsnapped the tourniquet, and said, "We're ready."

Ever so slowly he pressed the plunger and the injection began. About a minute later, with most of the drug still in the syringe, the patient gasped, made a series of gurgling sounds, and died. There was simply no way to miss it. Dave carefully placed the alcohol sponge over the vein, withdrew the needle, and walked to the foot of the bed. He handed the syringe to the instructor and said to the horrified students, "Well, girls, that's show biz," and left. He barely made it back to the ward before the Chief of Medicine was demanding he come to his office immediately. It was a close call, but he wasn't canned.

About a week into my Pediatrics rotation, I was dropped by a ripping case of chicken pox. I was in bed for week and off for another. That took care of my two weeks of vacation time. Yes, illness was deducted from vacation time.

Just before Pediatrics, I received word I had passed the Public Health Service exam and was accepted if I wanted to join. In exchange for covering me for a day, I took a weekend day for another intern, and went to the Army Office of Recruitment in Washington, DC. I hadn't yet received my draft notice, told the recruiter about the PHS option, asking if there might be something more enticing the Army could offer.

He was ready for it, and opened with something like, "Well, don't be too quick to reject a tour in Vietnam."

"No thanks."

"Well, Korea is amazing at this time of year, and the food…"

"No thanks."

"Have you ever been to the Philippines?"

"How about something closer to home?"

"The Old Soldiers Home here in the city has an opening…"

"Not really."

"Okay, then try this: the Pentagon is a great place to be. It's busy, exciting, and the Dispensary is right on the mall. No inpatients, and you only see officers."

"Interesting. Anything else?"

"Yes, well, there is one other possibility: Fitzsimons Hospital in Aurora, Colorado, has a place for a General Medical Officer."

Aurora?! My wife and I had just discussed living out west if I went with the PHS. We were already primed.

"I'll take it!" I signed on the dotted line and went home with the good news. Fitzsimons would give me inpatient and outpatient experience in an enormous, up-to-date hospital, lots of support, a chance to start a career path—all of it in the shadow of Denver. We were excited! What could go wrong? He promised me the position. Pack the bags.

Of course, I still had to finish the internship, pass Part III of the National Boards, and get my license, but the sudden reality of moving west gave me a surge of energy and confidence.

I had two months of OB-GYN coming up, something I imagined to be a lot like surgery only with even more sleepless nights.

The residents were universally positive, non-threatening, and like the surgeons, had a strong "Do One" ethic. While they provided great cover, we were expected to be able to handle prenatal care, routine deliveries, and D&Cs on our own.

I was quickly introduced to something I hadn't seen at all in medical school: the BOA birth. "Born on Arrival" applies to cases of a patient delivering just as she arrives at the hospital. It happened surprisingly often, especially with patients who had not had any prenatal care. It was usually a wild scene with a patient in the last moments of labor, panicked relatives—often with kids—and emergency people, all tangled together in the craziness of the moment. It was especially daunting for patients in the waiting room when the circus swept through.

I didn't have long to wait, either. On my first night in the OB reception area, a man rushed through the door yelling for help. His wife had given birth in their truck, and they couldn't find the baby! Nurses grabbed a "BOA Kit"—always at the ready—and we rushed outside. In the truck, an obese woman was rolling around the seat screaming she had lost her baby. Her pants were halfway off, tangled in her bloomers, all of it covered with blood. We could hear the sounds of a baby, apparently lost somewhere inside the bloomers. First we found the placenta, and following the umbilical cord, we found the baby alive and well, stuck in one of the leggings. Everything was untangled, the mother and child were admitted, and the husband was given what he needed to clean up the truck.

There was one recurring, rarely discussed controversy to deal with: abortion. It wasn't legal, and people had strong feelings about it. Some things don't change. Still, there were many women who sought abortion, and for them, there were limited options. The well-heeled found sympathetic physicians who masked the procedure as a "D&C," commonly done in the aftermath of a miscarriage. For the poor, there was either a potentially deadly back room "operation," or being admitted to a hospital professing the symptoms of early miscarriage hoping a D&C would be prescribed by a sympathetic staff physician, usually with a knowing wink.

Several times I was assigned to do "D&Cs," sometimes under pretty close supervision, sometimes not—depending on how busy the resident was. The operating room was located just down the hall from the ward. The nurses usually helped me move the patient from her bed into the OR, but sometimes they stopped at the door, leaving me to struggle the patient onto the operating table alone. It was immediately clear many of the nurses wanted nothing to do with what they knew to be a poorly disguised abortion.

I had no personal objection, especially knowing that refusing a safe abortion in the hospital almost certainly meant a botched procedure elsewhere, and instead of seeing the patient for a day on the ward, we would see a seriously ill patient in the ER. So, I simply did as I was told. The residents were nearby, but I was essentially by myself. That meant I had to manage the tricky business of administering local anesthesia to control pain. When that couldn't be done, I did spinal anesthesia usually under the brief direction of an anesthesiologist.

It was dicey and uncomfortable, another situation with no reasonable way out beyond following what I had been taught, doing the best job I possibly could. I was very glad when that part of the rotation was over.

There is, however, one additional event to describe, its title: *John Jesus, Part Three. Conclusion.*

A woman pregnant with her eighth child was admitted in early labor. She was travelling, had received no prenatal care at home, and did not appear to be in robust health. She was taken to the delivery area, prepared, and an IV was started. She made it clear she didn't object to the IV as long as it was just sugar water, and did not contain any medication. That would have been against her religion, and she would rather die than go back on her promise to God and her church that she would never give in to the Devil's potions.

She was told her wish would be respected as long as everything went well; after all, she had delivered a number of times without drugs. Unfortunately, her uterus wasn't up to the task of another delivery, and after several hours of stalled labor, it was clear she needed either a caesarean or a dose of Pitocin, a synthetic hormone used to start or enhance uterine contractions. Its discovery in 1955 earned Vincent Vagnaud a Nobel Prize in chemistry.

The woman would have none of it. We all tried to persuade her, nothing worked, and she was getting worse by the minute. Of course, she had already ruled out a caesarian section. As we talked, I asked about her church, where it was, and what they preached. To my surprise, her church was in Philadelphia. When I asked her the name of her pastor she said, "John Jesus."

Doing my best not to look dumbfounded, I said I had gone to school in Philadelphia, and John Jesus was a personal friend. She was amazed, understandably doubtful, but said that if I got John on the phone, and he said it was all right, she would accept Pitocin in her IV. It didn't take long to reach the church, and miraculously, John Jesus himself.

"Hello, John," I said as if we had just talked last week, "This is Brother Philip from Jefferson..." Before I could get the "remember me?" part out, he said of course he remembered, and what could he do for Brother Philip? I explained the situation, said I knew just how passionate he and he parishioners were about the Word of God, but we just needed to add a tiny dose of a hormone—not some awful medication—to the IV to save two lives. John agreed, talked to the woman, and in a few minutes the Pitocin flowed, she delivered, and a couple of days later she and her baby left for Philadelphia. She promised to say hello to John for me.

[handwritten margin note: another good story]

That was my last contact with the amazing, enigmatic, passionate John Jesus. I tried hard to find out what happened to John, but everything was a dead end. Maybe someday the answer will pop up. It would be just like John to have it that way.

With just three and half months left, I returned to Internal Medicine, which was to include several weeks on the neurology service. When I arrived, two of us were assigned to a particularly difficult case of a woman we called Grace, a middle-aged, bed-ridden woman drifting in and out of awareness, the consequence of a host of problems, principally uncontrolled diabetes, severe obesity, and multiple enormous decubitus skin ulcers—"bed sores"—beyond anything any of us had seen before. Because it was so hard move her, she couldn't be rotated to minimize pressure on any one part of her body. No one wanted to go into the room, and anyone who did would first don a face mask soaked in oil of wintergreen.

The single most daunting task for us was trying to deal with the skin ulcers and infection that came with them. We had the daily task of debriding them; meaning, surgical work to keep them clean and dressed. I don't recall any relatives visiting Grace, and given her condition, we all hoped she would pass away, freeing her from her painful, delirious slow death.

Our Internal Medicine resident that month was the Great Gomez, who graciously shared the seemingly endless debriding chore with us. One day, after a particularly long stretch closed in the suffocating room, Gomez said to no one in particular, *"Ella no se cosina en dos aguas,"* *You couldn't cook her if you boiled her twice,* a rough version of, "It's hopeless," an unspoken feeling we all shared.

Our responsibility was to provide care, no matter the dim prognosis. When we were overwhelmed with the task, we called a surgical resident to undertake more aggressive debriding than we dared.

The surgeons hated it. They told us to be more assertive, and implied that maybe a little push would solve the problem once and for all. One day, responding to yet another consultation request, an angry resident showed up with a syringe and a bottle of medication in his hand. He said it was time to do something about the situation, went into the room, and closed the door. About fifteen minutes later he emerged, said the patient had died, and left.

Grace was indeed dead, and while the staff seemed relieved to be done with the cruel and seemingly pointless exercise of keeping Grace alive, the two of us were in a dilemma. We thought the resident had probably given the patient a lethal dose of morphine, but we didn't see it, and had no way to confirm it. After talking it over with Gomez, following his recommendation, we went to the head of our department.

It was beyond uncomfortable. The Chairman asked a lot of questions, established that while it certainly appeared to be euthanasia, it was equally true the patient was already on the razor's edge of death, and we had no proof of wrongdoing. Finally, he thanked us for bringing it to his attention, and said he would take it up with the Dr. Hume.

That was the last we heard of it. We went back to work, and I was glad to move on to neurology. But images of Grace have never faded.

Neurology was a totally different discipline from anything else in the internship, distinct even from its close relative, Internal Medicine, far closer to medical art than anything I had seen before. Neurology is like a good detective story, a Nero Wolfe puzzler involving the nervous system. You follow the clues through a logical sequence based on the history of the illness and findings of the neurological examination. With that, you can pinpoint the location of the problem, and solve the mystery. We didn't have the scans and other diagnostic tools available today to confirm or challenge our conclusions, but the logic and sequence of figuring out where in the nervous system the problem arises remains unchanged.

It was also the most collegial of all the disciplines I had seen up to that point. The staff would gather, drink coffee, smoke their pipes, and talk through cases. I don't know why, but there were more pipes in evidence in neurology and psychiatry than any other specialty. Maybe it's the pace, maybe the nicotine sharpens cognition—who knows?

My early enthusiasm was tempered somewhat when I realized that a neurology practice has two distinct disadvantages. First, in the work outside of a teaching hospital, not every case is a mystery; far from it, there is a lot of repetition, especially headaches and seizures. Secondly, treatment plays a disappointing role. There were, and are, protocols for treating most neurological disorders, but conditions like MS, stroke, ALS, and many more are simply beyond effective care. The hackneyed phrase "Great Strides" applies to acute stroke management, and some other conditions, but treatment for the vast majority of chronic conditions remains frustratingly weak.

The last two months were in the ERs, starting with the pell-mell world of the Black ER. It was immensely gratifying to be able to apply what I had learned over the past year to the multitude of problems we faced day and night. Happily, too, medical residents were there all the time, and surgical support was instantly available. The place ran at top speed with amazing efficiency.

The last month, fortunately, was in the relative ease of the white ER. That gave us time to pack up and prepare to move temporarily to San Antonio, Texas, to join the Army Medical Corps for five weeks of indoctrination before being dispatched to Colorado. I had my license, but the question of what specialty might be best was still unresolved. It didn't really matter; after all, two years of Army medicine and life in the Wild West would surely make the answer obvious.

Then came the unanticipated case that changed everything.

It was late in the evening, there were no patients at all in the ER, and I was sitting at the desk with a nurse and a psychiatry resident drinking coffee, talking about nothing much. I had gotten to know Dr. Rothermel through his friend, Alan Cohen, and he often dropped by to chat, especially if Alan was there. Rothermel was a dramatic-looking man, tall and dark, with a black eye patch over one eye.

We heard a distant siren and waited for the Doppler effect to tell if it was coming to us, or turning off to the other ER. It was coming our way, and a few minutes later, even before the doors opened into the ER proper, we heard screaming—clearly a woman in a lot of pain. The doors burst open, and two attendants pushed an ambulance gurney into the room. An elderly woman clutched her chest, writhing in pain, yelling, "My heart! My heart!" The nurses moved her onto a bed, pulled the curtain to ready the patient for examination, and I stood up ready to go to work.

Rothermel was grinning. "Want to give me a consult?" Meaning, would I sign a yellow consult form formally asking him to evaluate the patient.

I was startled, thought something disdainful about psychiatrists, and told him to stand aside—let a *real* doctor deal with the apparent heart attack. The woman's distress did not let up, but we were able to get her vital signs (low BP, high pulse, panting respirations), observe her pale nail beds (anemia), mildly clubbed fingers (nonspecific; often heart or lung disease), and wrinkled skin (from dehydration). Next, an EKG and chest x-ray were attempted, both disrupted by the patient's agitation and constant movement. I started an IV and ordered lab work, looking particularly for elevated enzymes associated with heart attack.

The chest x-ray seemed clear, what could be seen of the EKG looked surprisingly normal, her BP held, but her agitation continued. Rothermel again asked if I wanted a consult? No! Just wait till you see the enzymes! But that was also a dead end. No hard evidence of a heart attack, but it could be early. Finally, I caved in, thinking either I'd show him, or he'd show me. Let's settle it.

He walked over to the bed, closed the curtain behind him, and thirty seconds later the moaning stopped. Fifteen minutes later, he opened the curtain revealing the patient sitting on the edge of the gurney, quietly talking to the psychiatrist. He handed her a card and said rather louder than need-be, "I'll see you next Tuesday." The IV was removed, and the patient left with a hospital attendant who gave her a ride home.

Okay, I was defeated, but curious. What had I missed, where did I go wrong?

"For starters, do heart attack victims usually make so much noise?"

"No, but so what—it's painful!"

"Aren't they usually really short of breath?"

"Yeah, but did you try to count her respirations? Who's to say she wasn't short of breath?"

"It's hard to keep screaming when you're short of breath."

"Not if you're panicked enough."

"Maybe," he said. "How about her socio-economic status?"

"Poor. Unkempt, unhealthy looking, probably doesn't get regular care. Just the sort of person prone to heart attack."

"True. Who was with her?"

"Nobody."

"Exactly. What about her hand?"

"Her hand? Well, she was anemic…"

"No, I mean what could you see from where we were? Left hand."

I was stumped, what was he driving at?

"A wedding ring."

"So?"

"So, what impoverished, debilitated, married woman goes *anywhere*, especially at eleven o'clock at night, without her husband? It doesn't happen. So, I simply got her to look at me, and asked, 'How long has he been gone?' She told me, 'Two weeks.' I told her I know how awful that pain is, we talked a while, and I'm going to follow up with her in the clinic."

It was a humbling experience. I needed to get knocked off my perch. Having survived the internship intact, license to practice in hand, and a new life out west about to start, it was good fortune to get taken down a few notches; even better, forced to consider an entirely new career track.

I always thought I was a good observer, the key to proper diagnosis. But the Rothermel experience made me think I was only observing what I wanted to see, not opening myself to the big picture. Wasn't that what neurology was about? It occurred to me that while I was licking my wounds over the Part II surgery disappointment, I hadn't noticed that my best test scores were in psychiatry, the result of not paying a lick of attention to any course work or textbook, but memorizing the highly condensed 1952 *DSM (Diagnostic and Statistical Manual)*, an effort that only took a couple of days, but its tight descriptions of all then-current psychiatric diagnoses cut through endless circumlocution, straight to the point. Clearly, I needed to augment my thinking and realize there were more options than Internal Medicine or its variations.

The internship ended with the last shift on Wednesday, June 30, and I was due at Fort Sam Houston in San Antonio, 1,500 miles away in Texas on July 1. Luckily, I found a resident willing to take most of my last shift, went home, took a brief nap, said goodbye to my family, and started the non-stop drive to Texas.

Twenty-three sleepless hours later, I joined 1,400 other weary, just-finished interns and residents at Fort Sam's Medical Field Service School to begin five weeks of training. At least this time around there was no morgue or any preparation agenda. It was a totally level (and deadly hot) playing field. Not one of us had any idea what was next. I certainly didn't know it would include performing surgery on a goat, crawling around a fake battlefield with bombs going off and bullets whizzing overhead, and through a total twist of good luck, find my career path. But it happened. Welcome to United States Army Medical Corps!

5

THE NEXT ADVENTURE

EXCEPT FOR A FEW QUICK naps, I drove straight through to San Antonio, arriving in time to join one of several consecutive waves of newcomers being herded into a large gymnasium to fill out papers, my introduction to the Army's ability to move large numbers of people in near-perfect synchrony.

Inside, there were hundreds of study hall desk-chairs arranged in perfect rows, each with a small writing surface hosting a stack of forms, and a sharp #2 pencil placed as precisely as the chairs. A loudspeaker voice told us over and over to take a seat, refrain from talking, and *DO NOT TOUCH THE PAPERS OR THE PENCIL!* Uniformed monitors circulated to be sure no one broke the rules.

It sounds ominous in the telling, and while certainly not friendly, or even superficially welcoming, it was clearly efficient. This is how you get 1,400 men, several hundred at a time, to complete numerous forms with the absolutely certainty that at the end, there would be no mistakes or need for correction. Nor could anyone possibly have a question or be confused. No matter how obvious, every single box was explained several times before we were told to pick up the pencil. After filling in a block, the same voice commanded: "Put the pencil down!"

Within four hours of arriving, I had registered, filled out a raft of forms, attended a lecture on precisely what was in our information kit, what the weekend reading assignment was, when and where we were to go on Friday to be fitted and to pay for our uniforms, where to get the many metal insignia for the uniforms, and when and where to go to get our immunizations. In any other universe, it would have taken a week to accomplish, but not in the Army. By Saturday afternoon, we had done all of it, leaving a little over a day to find an apartment so my family could join me for five weeks in what felt like the hottest city in the country. Happily, there was a large bulletin board in the mess hall filled with information about every imaginable service, including available housing, along with cost and directions. By Sunday afternoon, I had found a two-room apartment in a large, two-story converted motel about twenty minutes south of Fort Sam. It looked ideal. The place was modern, clean, affordable, sported a big pool and a cheerful front office. What I didn't notice was the fact it was located near Lackland Air Force Base, and that almost the entire place was filled with Air Force personnel, both active-duty airmen and contractors. In fact, we were the only Army family in the entire place. So what? So plenty, it turned out. I had no idea about the intense—sometimes nasty—rivalry between the services, a situation we quickly had to address.

The next surprise was just how fast our uniforms were ready. By midweek, we were properly suited, had been divided into two battalions, each divided into companies, platoons, and squads. The platoon was our basic training unit, itself made up of four squads of 10 men each. Every morning, well ahead of sunrise, everyone gathered in sleepy formation on the large parade ground in the center of the Field School.

Why so early? Because we had to learn to march, and if we waited for sun-up, it would quickly become too hot to march. As always, the Army had an answer, a scaled combination of temperature, humidity, and dew point dictating when it was safe to march.

Imagine taking 1,400 physicians whose only prior exposure to marching was watching their school band tromp around a football field at halftime, get them up at 4:00 a.m., dress them in a coat and tie uniform, assemble them in the dark, shout unintelligible commands at them, and expect they would somehow learn to move in perfect synchrony through a series of starts, stops, and turns of various sorts.

Impossible, even for the Army. We were constantly running into each other, turning the wrong way, taking too many or too few steps, and never—absolutely never—were we able to stay in a straight line either horizontally or vertically. It was like the cast of *Stripes* rehearsing in the dark. And we never really got any better. By sunup, the best we could do was somehow line up one arm's length from each other and stand at attention until given the "Parade Rest" command. That meant feet slightly apart, hands clasped behind your back, eyes on the commanding officer.

Once we were in formation, there was a seemingly endless roll call. Hearing your name triggered an immediate, "Present, Sir!" in a loud voice, with strong emphasis on "Sir!" When that was done, we were inspected; actually, our uniforms were inspected. The position of every insignia was measured, and corrections stopped the entire process. We quickly learned to get that part absolutely right, and not be the fool who held us up because his chrome Lieutenant's bar was crooked. Finally, notices were read out, and we were dismissed to start class at 8:00 a.m. sharp.

That routine was changed about a week into the process when platoon commanders showed up with a clutch of envelopes, and after roll call, handed them out one at a time. A name was called out, the man marched up, saluted, took the envelope, and returned to his place trying hard to make the turns sharp, and land the last two steps so he was dead even with the line. After we were dismissed, we found out the envelopes contained change-of-order notices. Whatever your initial assignment, it was out the window. Even worse, while a few were for Korea, almost all of the rest were for assignments in Vietnam.

It was the dread of dreads. There was no appeal, no questioning it. Holy shit! That changed every morning from a romp with the Keystone Cops into a terrifying suspense experience. If your name was called, you had to stand there with the unopened envelope under your arm, sweating from anxiety and the rapidly rising temperature.

Sure enough, in the middle of the second week my name was called. After I got back in line, I stood there trying to imagine what I would tell my wife, and where in the world they would go while I was in a jungle war zone eight thousand miles away. And, yes, there was a lot of anger, too. The bastards made a promise! Why didn't I play it smart and stay with the Public Health Service?

It took only a few seconds after hearing, "Dismissed!" to learn my fate: the Army Dispensary at the Pentagon. It wasn't Vietnam or Korea, but it sure wasn't Colorado, either. But at least they gave me my second choice, the honorable way to make the change. Clearly, it could have been a lot worse.

Every day was filled with classes starting with learning Army regulations, including a line-by-line study of *Customs and Traditions*, an incredibly detailed manual covering everything from where you stand in any particular situation to how to get in and out of a car, where you sit in a car, when you can leave a gathering if senior officers are present, even how your required calling card is to be printed: scripted or shaded Roman print. On that last point, a new rule: engraving was no longer required—simple printing would do. Wives were also required to have a calling card, just her name, no initials allowed. We were also admonished to live within our means, and above all, remember that "Vulgar speech is inexcusable," and "Excessive food or alcohol is boorish."

There was an entire section for our wives to study, starting with a bibliography referencing ten books and manuals conveniently for sale at the post book department or at the post library. Suggestions included *Etiquette* by Emily Post, *Complete Book of Etiquette* by Amy Vanderbilt, plus a few spellbinders like *Etiquette and Protocol*, and *The Army Wife Today*.

Next, an entire section titled, "Guidelines for Hemlines," embracing details for Morning Dress, Early Afternoon Dress, Late Afternoon Dress, Early Evening or Cocktail Dress, Dinner

Dress, and, of course, Dinner-dance Dress. Study hard, and don't forget: a hat and gloves are required for proper Early Afternoon Dress.

A few quotes:

"The first requirement of an Army wife is adaptability."

"She must learn Army standards and requirements so she may understand problems faced by her husband."

"She must be a good manager and always neighborly."

"By her patient understanding, zealous loyalty, and infinite resourcefulness, she adds grace and charm to her life and the whole military family."

My wife choked over that last one, but she was gradually getting used to Army-Think. What she wasn't getting used to, however, was the aloof treatment she and young Philip were getting at "home," especially at the pool, by Air Force wives. The kids mingled, but otherwise, she was left alone. Something had to be done.

After talking it over, we decided the best answer was the boldest. We bought a large toy truck, wrapped it in birthday paper, put it in a box along with a card, wrapped the box in brown paper with carefully knotted cordage—the way packages were sent in those days—and in bold letters, addressed it to ourselves with the return address of General and Mrs. D.D. Eisenhower at their farm in Gettysburg, Pennsylvania. We wrapped that package and sent it to a friend in Maryland who took it to Gettysburg and mailed it back.

Packages were delivered to the front office and placed on a table near the door for pickup by residents. You could see the table through the window, and my wife watched for the package to show up. When it did, she waited until there were quite a few people in the office, took Philip by the hand and walked in. She went to the mailbox, seemingly unaware of the package. The manager told her there had been a delivery, and with everyone watching, she picked up the package.

"Oh, look! Godfather didn't forget your birthday after all!"

Philip was excited, didn't give a fig who it was from or why, and had the whole thing open in seconds. He was thrilled with the truck, and we were thrilled with the sudden thaw in the social ice at the South New Braumfels Avenue Apartments.

Learning about saluting and the fundamentals of Army rules quickly gave way to learning about war; specifically, the diseases and wounds one would have to be prepared to deal with in just a few weeks. Not just malaria, yellow fever, and typhoid, but parasites, snake bite, jungle rot, and devastating bullet wounds, all of it only vaguely familiar to us. And what better way to get started than the Goat Course?

This section will be tough reading for some, but it describes an effective training method no one questioned at the time. Back in physiology class we did experiments on live dogs, animals that were sacrificed after we were finished. It would never happen today, of course, but at the time, it felt like this was simply what one did to prepare for dealing with patients.

The Goat Course was held in an enormous tent, a vast area filled with tables; on top of each one, a wounded goat. The goats had been anesthetized, shot in the upper leg, brought in, and laid out for us to practice bleeding control and wound debridement, the process I described in the story of caring for Grace. We did our work supervised by a few Army surgeons and the many surgical residents in our group. We also did the same cut-downs and intubations that I described earlier when one of our patients died. After we were finished, the goats were sacrificed.

Next came another encounter with something approximating the battlefield, this time a three-day assignment at Camp Bullis, a desert training facility north of San Antonio. We were sent in groups, so we were pre-warned of what to expect by others who had already had the Bullis experience. Frankly, I looked forward to it, a nice break from repetitive classwork—and a chance to leave coat and tie behind.

Training started with practice setting up a field hospital. Trucks unloaded crates of supplies, tents were erected, tables, beds, and an OR were all set up. Then helicopters came in with "patients" whose fake wounds, blood-soaked bandages, and needleless IVs looked like the real thing. It was *M*A*S*H* without the humor. (I know, the book was two years later, the TV series five, but the comparison holds).

As always, what initially looked and sounded like chaos quickly became order. Instructions shouted over the din were quickly obeyed. Afterward, it was all taken down, carefully stored, trucks and helicopters left, and our performance was reviewed. We moved on to another task, and the drama played out again for the next group.

We were housed in tents in groups of two squads each. Everyone was exhausted by the end of the day, but not enough to stop a lot of complaining. Clearly, these were not people who liked getting dirty. If they had ever gone to camp, it had been some sort of sanitized tennis camp or an overnight in a cabin with a hot shower and a ceiling fan. This was not the hunting and fishing crowd I was used to.

But what really got them upset was the idea of going to the rifle range to qualify on the M1 Garand rifle. Most had never fired a gun in their lives and were terrified it would kick their teeth out. Wasn't there some way they could skip the whole thing? "I'm a doctor, for God's sake! I'm never going to shoot anybody!"

I told them the kick was not the least bit unpleasant—my attempt to be helpful. They wanted to know how I knew such a thing. "Because I have one," I said. "I've been shooting all my life. I bought an M1 when I was in college. It's one of my favorite rifles." My colleagues looked at me like I was a leper. "Oh, and don't forget: we have to go through the infiltration course, too. Live bullets, right over our heads. We have to do again it at night, too, remember?" I couldn't help myself.

The next day, after more running around in the dust in different field hospital set-ups, we went to the rifle range. The instructions were exactly like perfect-pencil-time in the gym, only this time it was a rifle and an eight-shot clip filled with high powered bullets.

Every step was outlined in painful repetition, and the few who dared to say they didn't want to do it at all were quickly told to shut up and listen. No exceptions.

Once we were on the line, and told to commence firing, I fired my eight shots, put the gun down as instructed, and waited for the range master to come over, check my position, and look downrange to see if I had hit anything.

"You shot too fast," he said dismissively. He looked through his scope, paused, and said, "You've done this before." I was told to stay put while he turned his attention to a man two spots down from me who hadn't fired a shot. He was terrified of the gun, and nothing the sergeant said would make him do it. He moved the man to my position, took me to his, and said, "Qualify him." I was happy to do it.

That left the infiltration course, the famous military training exercise designed to get recruits as close to battle conditions as possible. The course is wider than it is long, allowing literally hundreds of soldiers to crawl across a simulated no-man's land at the same time. Our course was about 75 yards from the deep trench on the starting side to the exit trench on the other. Several control towers loomed over the entire field on the exit side, allowing spotters to watch for problems like men getting hopelessly tangled in the barbed wire obstacles, or worse: standing up. A row of machine guns stared across the field, fired electronically from the tower. There were dozens of circular pits in the course containing explosives, also detonated electronically from the tower. There was barbed wire everywhere, the challenge being to crawl along on your belly, and when you came to a tangle of wire, get on your back, push the wire up, and slide under. Going under on your belly won't work.

The machine guns were fixed in position to allow some travel side-to-side, but no change in elevation up or down. The fact the bullets and tracers pass above the height of a standing soldier is easily forgotten as you crawl through nettles and cactus quills, explosions going off all around, dust and dirt constantly falling on you, and the incessant rattle of the machine guns making it feel like the bullets were ripping by just inches over your head. It's even more dramatic at night, especially when you flip over on your back and see the tracers burning through the dust just above you.

My feeling about doing the infiltration course was one of excitement. Here was a chance to experience something utterly unique, never to be forgotten. My comrades were far less sanguine. A few were curious, but most were stuck between resentful and just plain afraid. Strangely, the thing they were most upset about was nettles, small land urchins that ignored clothing and went straight into the flesh, especially around knees and elbows. Others who had already done the course had quite a bit to say about nettles, so much so that many came equipped with the ultimate nettle armor: Kotex pads. It was a stunning sight, men wrapping sanitary pads around their elbows and knees, secured with adhesive tape, concealed under their clothing. They walked like zombies, but clearly thought they had outflanked the enemy.

It didn't work. In the first ten yards of crawling, all of the protection was pulled away, some of it left sticking out of sleeves and trouser legs. In the end, we all got equally nettled.

We marched to the field, filed into the rear trench, and waited for the command to start crawling. Instantly, there was a huge amount of noise from machine guns, explosives going off, people yelling, all of it going on in what seemed like a dust storm. Still, you could glimpse the towers, and thus know which direction to crawl, but berms around explosion pits and tangles of barbed wire prevented travel in anything approaching a straight line.

We had barely gotten started when suddenly everything stopped, the loudspeakers told us all to hold our positions, and to my right, there was a lot of excited yelling. One of our number had snapped and stood up! Within seconds a group of soldiers had picked their way through the wire, hoisted the man up, and taken him back to the trench. Within two minutes it all started again.

At one point, perhaps halfway through, someone crawled up next to me at panic speed, started to go under several strands of wire without turning over—and promptly got stuck. I did him the favor of lifting the wire so he could get through, expecting he would turn around and return the favor. No way. All I saw was the soles of his boots heading for the exit.

We tumbled into the exit trench, pulled a lot of nettles out of our clothes, and were marched back to camp. That night, we did the whole thing again. This time no one stood up, and no one bothered with the padding. The lack of light wasn't as much of a problem as I had expected. The towers were lighted, and feeling wire against your helmet told you when it was time to flip over.

The final trial was the tear gas house, a fake house with a dirt floor, filled with tear gas. We were up at our usual 4:00 a.m., marched to the house to stand in a very slow line to our destination. There was a lot of grumbling in the line, best summed up by a dermatologist, Joel Wilentz, who said: "All my life I lived in New York City, and they get me up in the middle of the night to tell me what gas smells like!"

When it was our squad's turn, we donned our gas masks, marched into the house, forming a line in front of an officer and two sergeants. We were instructed to step forward one at a time, stand in front of the officer, remove the gas mask, salute, state our name, rank, and serial number, slowly in a loud voice, and wait until the officer returned the salute and said, "Dismissed!" Then one was allowed to replace the mask, do one of those, it-never-worked-spin-around-reverse moves, and leave. Outside, there was water to wash away the tears and stinging residue.

Back in San Antonio, with just two weeks to go, my wife and I were getting used to the idea of living in the Washington area, though the part about working in a purely outpatient clinic was disappointing. I had hoped the wider exposure to practice options at Fitzsimmons Hospital, plus life in the Wild West, would solve the specialization riddle. But as always, the answer was closer at hand than I had imagined.

After lunch one day, while scanning the bulletin board, a notice announcing a meeting for psychiatrists caught my eye, an invitation to an informal get-together to discuss—among other things—a five-month "OJT in Psychiatry." How odd. What interest would a group of post-residency psychiatrists have in On the Job Training? I decided to go—just curious.

About thirty psychiatrists, many who already knew each other, gathered along with the Chief of Service, Colonel Jones, and his deputy, Colonel McGonagal, Director of Chambers Pavilion, the post's in-patient psychiatric hospital. I sat in the back waiting for some mention of the OJT, but the meeting droned on about the rules of military psychiatry, and the role each would play in battlefield conditions, all of it without a word about OJT. It would have been disrespectful to leave, so I sat, daydreaming, until the end. As the meeting was about to break up, Colonel Jones asked if there were any questions, so I raised my hand to ask if there might be some information about the OJT program?

I expected a simple yes or no, not the reaction I got. The Colonel and his assistant looked at each other, and said quite clearly, "Oh, no!" All thirty of the psychiatrists looked at me disparagingly, there was some mumbling, the colonel excused the group, and told me to come forward. It was beyond awkward, and I immediately apologized for whatever it was that so upset the meeting. I was told that the "problem" I presented was not my fault. It seems the Army was doing away with the OJT program, but the rules forced at least a last attempt to fill the one remaining, absolutely last ever, unfilled slot. Only then could it be officially shut down. Acceptance of any "qualified applicant" was also mandated, so realistically, they had to accept me if I wanted it. Weirdly, they seemed to be over a barrel, and needed to confer. I was told Colonel McGonagle, would be in touch.

I waited almost a week, completely unsure of what—if anything—was next. Meanwhile, we were getting ready for the move to Washington. But while in formation one morning, I got a note from Colonel McGonagel telling me to meet him in the Pavilion that afternoon.

Unlike the gloomy response at our first meeting, this time he was cheerful, and without really telling me anything about the "program," said I would be welcome to join the "staff" at Chambers after graduation the following week. The program would last five months, my orders would be changed so I could report to the Pentagon after finishing, and the training would help my career no matter where it went after the service.

I accepted, we extended our lease, and looked forward to staying put, having a chance to learn more about south Texas, plus giving us plenty of time to plan for the transition to Washington.

Graduation was over by midday on a Thursday. I proudly put on my brand-new Captain's bars, and headed for the hospital to meet Colonel McGonagle and his staff. It was puzzling that there was only one other officer in the colonel's office, Dr. Lawrence, like myself, freshly out of the Field School. He had completed his residency just weeks before, and his permanent duty station was Ft. Sam Houston. The colonel explained that Cambers Pavilion was an inpatient unit with four male wards of thirty men each, and a single female ward housing thirty women. So far so good, but where were the other psychiatrists?

Colonel McGonagle saved the best for last: it seems that there had been a sudden need for psychiatrists in the Vietnam arena, and his entire staff had just been transferred out. All four of them were gone.

"So, Captain Lawrence, you'll take two male wards, Captain Hirsh will take the other two, and I'll take the woman."

I was way past stunned. Dr. Lawrence was unhappy with the patient load. Are you kidding? I had landed in a zone where five patients would be too much. Dr. Lawrence was dismissed, taken off by his sergeant-assistant to meet his sixty patients and move into his new office. When they were gone, Colonel McGonagle told me he understood my situation, hoped I had some familiarity with psychiatry, and in particular, the use of psychiatric drugs. I said that basically, I didn't have a clue, and wondered if this whole thing wasn't a terribly bad idea. I was told there was no other option, I would do well to look like I knew what I was doing, study as much as possible, "And read this. It will help." He slid a copy of Harry Stack Sullivan's *The Psychiatric Interview* across the table, stood up, and offered to show me to my new office where I would meet my staff, the sergeants and mix of civilian and Army nurses who ran the wards.

"Oh," he said, almost as an afterthought. "We usually start at eight o'clock, but tomorrow is Friday, so be here at seven-thirty. It's your day to give shock treatment." Before I could say, "Are you CRAZY?!" he added: "Don't worry, the sergeant will help you."

The staff was obviously leery of the newcomer, especially when I was so vague about my prior experience. I told them an undated version of the Rothermel story, saying it was what propelled me into psychiatric training. Weak, I know, but it was the best I could do. Then we went to the two wards, each an enormous room with fifteen beds on each side of a center aisle. There were no curtains between the beds, no privacy at all.

When we walked in, everyone rushed to the foot of his bed and stood at attention. I gave my first-ever "At Ease," hoping it sounded like something I did ten times a day. Introductions were made, and we left. I spent the rest of the afternoon studying charts, carefully writing down two things: diagnosis and medication. I was shown where to go to give the shock treatments, wondering how in the bloody world I was going to pull that one off without hurting anyone, or getting in a heap of trouble.

It was pointless to go to the post library and imagine getting any helpful text to study, so I drove home, tried to explain the situation to my bewildered wife, and spent half the night reading about how a renowned, eccentric psychoanalyst conducted an interview. There was nothing there about shock treatment or medication.

The next morning, I marched in with all the confidence I could muster. There, seated in a hallway by the treatment room, were eight pajama-clad soldiers, all of them seemingly non-apprehensive. I said, "Good morning," with all the calm nonchalance I could summon, and walked into the room. Inside, there were six corpsmen, a nurse, an anesthesiologist, and a Wise Old Sergeant. Obviously, Colonel McGonagle had clued him in, and he quietly led me to the ECT device, told me *sotto voce* to watch him, and when he nodded, rotate the "glissando switch" to cock the machine, and when he nodded again, push the black button. Simple.

Each man came in, got on the gurney, and an anesthesiologist injected two drugs: one to induce sleep, the other to momentarily paralyze the man's muscles. The purpose of the shock is to cause a seizure; without it, there is no benefit. But an unprotected seizure could potentially cause injury—broken bones and teeth—but with the muscles paralyzed, the seizure is barely visible, and there is no post-treatment discomfort. Within minutes, except for some transient memory loss, recovery is complete.

I pushed the button eight times that day, and many more over the next five months. Ironically, I was never allowed to do it in my residency—way too dangerous, they said. Didn't matter, I was already an expert.

With help from Dr. Lawrence, Colonel McGonagel, and the staff, I was able to begin absorbing the basic mechanics of my job, starting with the key elements in medication treatment; particularly, their potential for serious side effects. Over time, I learned better interviewing skills, as well as more confidence in the most daunting part: making an accurate diagnosis.

It also quickly became apparent I needed all my medical skills to avoid mistaking a physical illness for a psychiatric problem. Early on, my cautionary manta became: "It's organic until proven otherwise." In other words, approach every psychiatric diagnosis presuming a physical, reversible cause. It's a rule that saved my patients, and me, many times over the years.

Most of our patients came from the war zone, airlifted directly to Lackland AFB from "RVN," our shorthand for the Republic of Vietnam. Some were dropped off in the Philippines or at other hospitals along the way. We were the end of the line. The rest of our patients were soldiers stationed at Ft. Sam Houston, and its main hospital, the Brooke Army Medical Center.

The diagnosis "PTSD" did not become part of our official nomenclature until 1980. The then-current equivalent was "Gross Stress Reaction" caused by "Combat or a Civilian Catastrophe." Because it was defined as both "transient and reversible," the goal of treatment was to help the soldier get back to duty with his unit as soon as possible.

When treatment was prolonged, the diagnosis shifted to "Neurotic Reaction," requiring a "more definitive diagnosis" to find a presumed underlying problem, something to explain why a simple thing like Gross Stress Reaction didn't resolve in a timely way. Unlike our understanding of PTSD today, at that time no consideration was given to the idea it could worsen over time, or that its onset could be delayed. Beyond providing a safe, nurturing environment, what we gave individually to patients was secondary to the salutary effect of the hospital milieu, a mix of support and pressure from peers, encouraging recovery coupled with the expectation of return to duty.

Today, PTSD is its own diagnosis, treatment is vastly more detailed, and derogatory implications are gone.

Our patient population was heterogeneous, a mix of disorders from multiple forms of psychosis and depression to personality disorders and malingering. We were also just awakening to the new, way under-recognized problem of drug abuse, especially hashish, heroin, and—yes—prescription drug dependence, through both street trade and prescription channels. Alcohol dependence seemed less prevalent. Enlisted men drank off base, usually in groups. For officers, the consequence of even simple public intoxication could be career-ending, and seeking help for dependence was completely off the table. On the battlefield, easily concealed pocket drugs were everywhere, allowed the user to keep shooting, and survive the horror going on around them. Better to die stoned than scared shitless.

There was one feature of our hospital population that hit me the minute I walked onto the ward: there were no officers, and my patients all looked like kids. The average age of the soldiers we treated was 18–21. No surprise, really. Remember, though the economy was humming along, in considerable measure because of spending on the war, it was a time when farming was falling away, technology was on the rise, and thousands of boys who barely struggled through high school were out on the street looking for work, especially in rural communities, where the best they were going to do was pump gas or work the night shift at the locker plant gutting chickens.

Many were caught in the draft; for others, there was enlistment. Recruiters dressed in snappy uniforms were everywhere offering jobs that came with pride, the promise of training during service, and free education after serving their country. Sign here, kid. In a few days, they were on a bus bound for basic training, and a few short months later, off to Southeast Asia to save us from the Commie hoards. Stick them in a rice paddy full of snakes and dead people, blow up everything and everyone around them, and see what happens.

Psychiatric illnesses like Schizophrenia and what we now term Bipolar Disorder, as well as many forms of depression, tend to reveal themselves late in the teen years and early twenties, pushed by a host of perturbations starting with genetic predisposition, the complex stress of leaving home, finding work, dealing with relationships, drugs—a deadly combination for a vulnerable emotional system. Imagine what happens to that predisposition in a combat situation. Again, it's easy to see why so many used drugs to numb the realization they could be dead any minute. It worked for some; it destroyed others.

Then there were the troublemakers, marginal kids who never really got along with authority, or worse: got in the service to stay out of jail. Many prosecutors pushed the service button as a quick way to clear out marginal cases. Surprisingly, some of those kids became great leaders. They were the ones whose rebelliousness and misbehavior weren't the product of an emerging antisocial disorder. When their fearlessness and aggression were channeled into leadership characteristics, they often did well.

But the budding antisocial kids were a huge headache. Quite a few were weeded out early in the game, discharged before they got into the mental health system. But many were clever, manipulative, and their cold, non-anxious way of thinking led them to game the system. Worse, they destroyed discipline and morale from the sidelines, almost invisibly. Their game was, "Hey! Let's you and him fight!" And while the fight was going on, they were laying down bets on the outcome.

I learned very quickly that when the ward milieu started to come unglued, it was rarely the hallucinating schizophrenic boy, or the withdrawn depressed soldier, causing the problem; no, it was the seemingly affable kid, the first one to leave just before the fight started.

About a month into my "training," just as I was starting to get a grip on the different forms of psychosis, an unusual patient was admitted, one who had been seen on a surgical unit at the main hospital by our Chief, Colonel Jones, found to be delusional, and was being transferred to my ward. Because of the man's unusual presentation, the Colonel would manage the case himself.

I was assured that because he was admitted as a trauma victim, a thorough diagnostic investigation had been conducted, ruling out any physical disorder, including alcohol withdrawal, that could be at the root of the problem. A psychotic reaction to anesthesia and surgery, while rare, was considered, though it is usually transient and not as severe as this man's paranoia. Even more mysterious: medication had not dented his condition.

When Mr. James arrived, I had another surprise: he was a Warrant Officer, a member of a special branch of the armed services positioned between enlisted troops and officers. They were a hybrid bunch, few in number, each with a specific technical or administrative skill set.

Because of the need for specialized nursing care, we arranged for the patient to be in a single room. His multiple bandages had to be monitored and changed frequently, plus he was unable to walk because he had a cast on each leg. He was groggy and inarticulate, presumably the consequence of a significant dose of Thorazine already started by the Chief. In spite of his mental fog, he was surprisingly animated, fearful, and overtly paranoid. The more he talked, the more bizarre it all sounded. He insisted his injuries were the result of being deliberately run down by espionage agents he had discovered trying to steal rocket secrets from a team of scientists from Huntsville, Alabama, temporarily stationed in San Antonio. True, his job description number did include intelligence work, but it seemed beyond belief he uncovered the plot, called the FBI, was told they would look into it, but fearing that would take too long, had started trailing the bad guys on his own. Late one night they spotted him, ran him down, and left him for dead. Really?!

While the story was beyond sketchy, there was no arguing both of Mr. James' legs were broken, he had a collapsed lung, and a host of cuts and abrasions. There was no family involved, his health record didn't contribute anything, and we were left with what appeared to be a delusional man whose injuries alone weren't likely to have caused such sudden, organized paranoia.

The Chief said he wasn't sure if this was a case of Paranoid Schizophrenia, a Paranoid Reaction—or something else entirely. He favored Paranoid Reaction.

This type of psychotic disorder is extremely rare. It is characterized by an intricate, complex, and slowly developing paranoid system, often logically elaborated after a false interpretation of an actual occurrence. Frequently, the patient considers himself endowed with superior or unique ability. (*Diagnostic and Statistical Manual of Mental Disorders*, 1952; changed only slightly in the *DSM* of 1968).

So what was it? As the dose of Thorazine rose, Mr. James became increasing garbled, but he stuck to his story. A week into his care, one could hardly understand him, though his fear of being in the hospital persisted. No amount of reassurance about security, guards, and alert soldiers made any difference.

One morning as I entered the building, the sergeant on duty told me there were two men waiting to see me in my office. Indeed, I was greeted by two grim-faced men in dark suits who flashed FBI badges and said, "You have one of our informants in your hospital. We are going to move him this morning." And they did. I have no idea what happened to Mr. James, but the effect on the rest of us was profound, starting with Colonel Jones.

To his credit, the colonel insisted on a thorough review to see where we had gone wrong. We all agreed the lack of any historical information had forced us to rely solely on the clinical appearance. The conversation seemed to veer off at that point into a rationalization of our failure based on the simple conclusion the man's story was too absurd not to be delusional. At that point, the military equivalent of Dr. Rothermel—Colonel McGonagal—stepped in. Like the rest of us, he had been sidelined by his boss, but when I privately shared my concern about the high doses of Thorazine, his cautious, middle-ground advice was to see how it played out.

While the "autopsy," as the review was termed, droned on, Colonel McGonagal sat in the corner, tipped back in his chair with a half-smile, half-smirk look of bemusement on his face. When it was his turn to talk, he started by saying that in his experience, the content of a delusion is rarely a good measure of the illness. The more important issue is how the delusion is presented, starting with the basic element of speech as a reflection of thinking. And what about his affect, his emotional tone? Each illness has its own patterns, don't skip the basics to focus on content.

He went on matter-of-factly to point out that in spite of agitation and the side effects of Thorazine, his speech flowed in a sequential way. Most importantly, his affect was appropriate to the content, even if the content seemed insane, an important characteristic of schizophrenia where there is typically a disconnect between the frightening nature of the delusion, and the patient's actual emotional response. He suggested we should have paid more attention to background and basics, and less to the dazzling nature of Mr. James' bizarre tale.

"We screwed up." That was it. There was really nothing else to say except we owe Mr. James an apology. For me, it was another lesson moment to add to my mental textbook: trust your doubts, doubt your assumptions, and treat carefully—especially when response is poor. Another axiom: no dose of medication can cover a faulty diagnosis.

Not long after the Mr. James episode, Colonel McGonagal called me into his office to ask about a particular patient, Gary G. His interest seemed puzzling. There wasn't anything particularly remarkable about Gary G., just a run-of–the-mill problem patient we were having trouble getting back to his unit. His symptoms were vague, but they had a peculiar habit of worsening every time discharge was mentioned. We recognized him to be a malingerer, but the issue was disposition, not diagnosis. His condition wasn't so blatant or his motive so clear he could be charged with anything; likewise, plenty of people advance symptoms consciously or unconsciously in reaction to stress. He wasn't disabled, yet getting him back to duty posed the risk of his acting out, either self-destructively or in a way that threatened unit cohesion.

Why was the Colonel asking? He showed me a letter, saying simply, "CI" as he slid it across the table. CI? I had never heard of that one.

"Congressional Interest," he explained, the result of a patient or his family taking a complaint or a grudge straight to the top. Skip the chain of command, the procedures, and reviews available for dealing with such matters. Screw that, write straightaway to your congressman. The letter complained that one of the congressman's constituents, a soldier bravely serving his country, was being deliberately deprived of his rights; specifically, the right to have visits with his wife. The congressman demanded an immediate investigation and remediation.

When I met Gary G. in my office, he had a copy of the letter in his hand, and a barely concealed look of triumph on his face. He didn't want to talk about the fact visits were never denied; no, he wanted to know what we were going to do about it now. I said it was simple enough: his wife was welcome to visit during any normal visiting hours. Not good enough. It turned out his wife was in north Texas, they didn't have the money for her to get to San Antonio, stay a day, and return home. He reminded me that the congressman expected action. The ball was in our court.

I was furious over being so manipulated, but as usual, Colonel McGonagel had the answer: we'll send a car, bring her to San Antonio, rent a motel room, and allow them a conjugal visit. Then send the bastard back to his unit and let his CO (commanding officer) handle it. We were done.

So it was. A car was sent, a motel room arranged, and the couple was allowed an afternoon reunion while two guards maintained vigil. Room service, however, was not included. After the visit, Gary G. returned to the ward, the envy of every other patient, and his wife was driven home. The colonel sent a flowery note to the congressman, and we started the discharge process.

Two days later, literally hours before Gary G. was to be sent back to duty, the ward sergeant came to me in a considerable state of agitation.

"Sir! We have a problem!" The ward was suddenly crawling with crab lice, and it hadn't taken long to figure out it was Gary G. who was the Typhoid Mary infecting Ward A1. Patients lived cheek by jowl with each other, showered together, sat on each other's bunks to talk—there were no chairs—the ideal petri dish for the spread of a rapidly growing population of hungry crabs.

All linen had to be cleaned, everything scrubbed, and everyone was twice treated with lindane, once to kill the current crop, the second time to catch any hatchlings. The place was on its ear, patients were agitated, staff stretched to the breaking point, all the while Gary G. sat scratching, wondering how in the world we could be blaming him.

A little digging revealed that Gary G. wasn't married, didn't come from north Texas, and had pulled off a spectacular scam, though in the end, it was his undoing. There was no psychiatric basis for his symptoms, and thus no justification for medical discharge, disability, or even continued treatment. He was sent back to his unit with a report about his lying, and the disruption it caused in carrying out our mission. Okay, Commander, it's your problem. My guess is Gary G. was summarily discharged.

We didn't see much of Colonel Jones after the Mr. James incident, reportedly because he was preparing to retire after 30 years of service. On his last day of making rounds with us, he demanded to know why one of my patients, a twenty-year-old boy with florid schizophrenic symptoms, had not been returned to his unit for duty. I pointed out the stubborn nature of his psychosis and lack of full response to medication, but the colonel wasn't impressed. He glared at me and said, "I don't give a damn if he sees Jane Mansfield on top of every filing cabinet, the question is: can he file?"

That soldier did not improve and was sent to a VA hospital for continuing care. He was given a medical discharge, "Line of Duty: Yes," meaning his illness occurred in the course of his duty, not the product of misbehavior, and thus the Army assumed responsibility for his treatment—no matter its duration. He would also receive ongoing outpatient care and disability income after he recovered.

I was unable to attend the Colonel's retirement ceremony because of the demands of my job.

As the end of my TDY (Temporary Duty) approached without any apparent change of orders, it seemed both safe and prudent to arrange for housing in the Washington, DC, area. I was allowed a quick leave, starting on a Thursday, to be back Monday morning. Using military transportation was free, flying commercial was expensive, so I opted to go to the Air Force Base with a transportation order, the only catch being scheduled flights to anywhere were a rarity. One had to fly the equivalent of stand-by. Early Thursday morning I was able to catch an early flight on a DC-3 going to DC. Slow but sure. What could go wrong? Settle down with a good book, study the real estate market.

About an hour out of San Antonio, we lost an engine, and had to make an emergency landing at Connally Air Force Base in Waco, Texas. That was bad enough; worse, there didn't seem to be any clear alternative to waiting to see if the crippled DC-3 could be fixed. About three hours into the wait, a four-engine plane stopped to pick up the Army Marching Band on its way to DC. Fantastic! I joined them. Other than making a couple of prolonged stops, everything was fine until we were about an hour past Nashville, when—you guessed it—we lost an engine, forcing us to turn back to the Nashville area. The pilot assured us we still had plenty of power to make a normal landing. Not to worry. But a few minutes later, we lost a second engine—on the same side as the first one. This time, the pilot wasn't quite as chipper. He said we still had enough juice to get back on the ground, but suggested we acquaint ourselves with the position used in an emergency landing. It was also clear the plane was losing altitude and dipping to the silent side. The changing pitch of the two remaining engines made it clear the pilot was having trouble keeping the engines synchronized. There was no helpful stewardess on board to coach or reassure us, just a handy folder next to the air sickness bag showing how to fold up like a theater seat to increase the chance of survival during a crash landing.

At that point, the band members who had instruments started playing "Abide With Me," and the rest sang. It was scant comfort, but at least a distraction. As we approached the field, the music stopped, we wrapped our arms around our legs, and held on during a wobbly but safe landing. Back in the terminal, I asked about the possibility of a flight to DC.

"Too bad, Captain. You just missed one. He's about to take off." Just in case it wasn't too late, he called the tower, the tower called the pilot who said if I got out there immediately, they'd take me. I was rushed into a jeep, driven like a drunken rodeo rider around the taxiways right to the end of the runway where a DC-3 just in from Waco was gunning its engines, ready for takeoff. The door opened, I got on the hood of the jeep, threw my bag in, and was pulled on board. Sure enough, it was the same DC-3 I left in Waco, repaired and ready to go.

I got into DC that night, and over the next two days saw a number of apartments, settled on an affordable townhouse in the Virginia suburbs, got back to the Air Force base, and on Sunday, hitched an uncomplicated ride back to San Antonio. Piece of cake.

It looked like smooth sailing from that point. With a week to go, we were told a new psychiatrist was coming to replace me. About the same time, I received another problem case, Carlo P., an American who went to Canada to avoid the draft, then weirdly joined the Canadian army, deserted, and fled back to the US. He was apprehended, put on a huge show of bizarre symptoms, and somehow ended up in Texas at our hospital. Once again, the question wasn't about psychiatric illness but about how to disentangle the man from the medical system into the legal system where he belonged.

Easier said than done. He immediately claimed to be hallucinating, threatened suicide—"To stop the voices!"—and turned the ward routine upside down. The new psychiatrist, recently returned from a tour in Vietnam, arrived in the middle of the Carlo P. disruption. Carlo had arrived on Monday, the new psychiatrist on Wednesday, and I was supposed to leave on Friday.

The new man was in a foul humor, having had no time off between his miserable RVN (Republic of Vietnam) experience and his new job in San Antonio. The last thing he wanted to deal with was an antisocial draft dodger masquerading as the victim of mental illness. After meeting Carlo, he decided the way to deal with him was to start ECT immediately, to "calm him down;" in other words, "shut him down." Even worse, since I was still on duty through Friday, ECT duty would fall on me.

I went to Colonel McGonagal begging for an ethical way out of the mess. As always, he thought for a while, then said I should check out of my TDY on Thursday, "Leave the rest to me." If the personnel at the check-out station questioned the exit time, he promised to cover me. I thanked him, and at the end of the day, I went home to start packing. My only remaining chore was to process out of Ft. Sam Houston.

It was a Thursday, and the check-out station was mercifully quiet. Two hours ought to do it, I reasoned, even if they have to get approval from the colonel. I stood in front of a corporal's desk for what seemed like an eternity while she sifted through my pile of official papers over and over. Finally, apologizing for the delay, she said there was a problem with my orders. Thinking it had to be the day-early issue, I prepared to refer her to the colonel.

But that wasn't the problem. It was my MOS, the number service members are given to describe their Military Occupation Specialty. There are literally hundreds of designations, each an extremely precise, super-condensed job description. My MOS was 3100, a General Medical Officer; meaning, I had completed my internship, thus qualified to do non-specialty, general medical work. It was the most basic MOS a physician could have, the utility infielder of the Medical Corps.

"A problem?"

"Yes, sir. Your orders say you are a 3100, but that's wrong: you're a psychiatrist, a 3129."

"Goodness," I said with mock seriousness, "How could that have happened?" I thought, of course, that when the idea of the TDY sank in, thoughts of being a fully trained, board eligible psychiatrist would fly out the window. But the corporal took it seriously, said she was terribly sorry for the delay, but it would take a while to go through and change my record, get it right. I didn't say anything, largely because I just wanted to get our lengthy road trip started, and also knowing that when I got to my duty station at the Pentagon, we could all have a good laugh over the mix-up. No big deal. I could enjoy my lofty status for a few days before getting back to reality.

The ride back was relatively easy, our new home in the wooded suburbs felt like a castle compared to six month's confinement in a two-room recovering motel in San Antonio. Suddenly, we had friendly neighbors, a community play yard, all within 20 minutes of the Pentagon. Nirvana!

There was no time to acquaint myself with the basics of the Pentagon before arriving for my first day of work. I knew that the place was enormous, had six zip codes, and that every day 25,000 people somehow found their way around its five concentric rings and myriad hallways. If you could lay the Empire State building on its side, point to point over the structure, only about 40 feet of its rooftop antenna would protrude.

Getting around depends on knowing the geographical guide code. The rings are lettered A–E, and office numbers are in clockwise sequence. It is said that in spite of its complexity, knowing the system, one can walk between any two points in fifteen minutes. There is a mezzanine on the second floor with shops and other services, and in the center, a park-like area, a quick way to stay connected to the outdoors.

Happily, the dispensary was located on the mezzanine just inside the south entrance. I was shown to the Chief's office where Colonel DelVeccio and his adjutant were waiting for me. I stood in front of the colonel's desk, saluted, announced I was reporting for duty, and handed my orders to the adjutant—as required by protocol. The colonel said he was delighted to "finally" see me, explaining the delay in my arrival had put quite a strain on their operation. He was interrupted by the adjutant.

"Sir! Look at this," he said pointing to the orders. The Colonel's happy face instantly disappeared.

"Jesus Christ! A psychiatrist! What the hell are they thinking?"

Recovering quickly, he said, "It's not you, Captain. It's just we had expected a GMO," [General Medical Officer] "not a psychiatrist." Before I could open my mouth to explain, he told me to wait in his outer office while he sorted it all out. I retreated, thinking he would make the necessary calls, the MOS mix-up would be repaired, and we could have that chuckle I had anticipated. When I was called back into the office, however, the Colonel was still grim-faced. Clearly, he hadn't made any calls. He again apologized for his outburst, then asked for a favor.

"A *favor*?"

"Yes," he said. "We've worked out an alternative solution." Would I be willing to take sick call every morning and provide psychiatric service in the afternoons?

"Certainly, sir. Anything to help," I said.

The Colonel and his adjutant seemed relieved, but I was instantly worried that my hutzpah would come back to bite me. But at that point, there was no turning back. "Let it ride," I thought. "See how it plays out." I was given an office, introduced to the other physicians and the dispensary staff. The two doctors who knew me—both from the Field School, one also from internship—didn't say a word about my status; in fact, it seemed to amuse them.

That was it. I was the Army's Pentagon psychiatrist, ready for work. "What the hell," I thought. My OJT experience had convinced me that a career in psychiatry was my most likely choice, and what could be better than a chance to test drive the idea without a commitment to buy, especially in such a hybrid place? If I got busted, I could plead ignorance; besides, the worst that could happen would be practicing general medicine for the next 18 months, a rabbit in the briar patch.

The dispensary was specifically for officers from all branches of the military service working in the building. It was not elitism but reflected the simple fact the Pentagon was the epicenter of the Department of Defense, home base for thousands of ranking officers. It was quite literally a base of its own, requiring the full range of base services, including medical support. The enlisted men and women stationed there were all members of units at nearby bases, each with its own medical resources. We had another function as well: we were the ER for the entire place.

Happily, the military men and women were all in good physical shape, a requirement of service, and unlike a town of 25,000, there were no children and hardly anyone over 65.

Still, we practiced emergency response regularly, taking turns on the "crash team," the equivalent of EMTs in an emergency vehicle today. Among our twenty physicians (including our CO) we had trained cardiologists, surgeons, internists, and a dermatologist, Dr. Wilentz, recovered from his experience in the gas mask exercise. Corpsmen and nurses were ready day and night with a rolling stretcher and a crash cart full of supplies. It is surprising how few times we actually had to deploy the team.

I quickly settled into the morning routine, but afternoons were a bit of a challenge, especially at first, before word spread that psychiatric consultation was available. I did my best to look busy, stay out of sight, and be as helpful as possible when I could. I took part in all of our training, the literature club, and our families often socialized.

Gradually, I started to get some business, though rarely an officer seeking personal psychiatric care. That could be a career-killer. Only a desperate situation would cause someone to take such a chance. In fact, I can recall only a handful who ever dared it, including a major who came to see me on a Tuesday afternoon, important to know because his problem had to be solved by Thursday afternoon. He had just been notified he was to ship out on Friday to a post in Texas, and from there, he was going to Vietnam.

His problem was a morbid fear of snakes, and from what he had heard, Texas and was crawling with snakes. He wasn't the least bit reassured by the reality that most snakes are harmless, and bad actors are seldom encountered; even then, they usually flee, and when they don't, they sound some sort of alarm. His fear was less about being bitten by a poisonous snake that idea he wouldn't be able to control his fear and be humiliated in front of his troops.

I was fairly well along at that point, my ample reading time having given me the chance to delve into a number of different treatment theories, including hypnosis and related interventions, such as using suggestion in motivated patients.

Without realizing it, the major had two powerful assets operating in his favor: he was highly motivated to overcome his fear and had vested me with near-mystical power to overcome his distress. My job was to take advantage of those assets.

"I can help you, but only if you agree to do exactly as I say. No questions, no protest, no modifications."

He accepted. I wrote the name "Arnie" and an Alexandria address on a card, instructed him to go to that address, and ask for Arnie. No hesitation, no backing out. Do it and you will be cured.

Okay, it was a wild move, but urgent situations sometimes require a truly out-of-the-box approach. I did everything I could to look utterly certain it would work, told the major there was no time or need for a follow-up appointment, and sent him on his way. As soon as he was gone, I called my friend Arnie, owner of a pet store heavily into tropical fish and—of course—snakes. I told him an Army major would soon show up, and I wanted him to be ready with a boa or some other docile snake, and when the man walked in, drop it around his neck.

"And if he has a freaking heart attack?"

Not to worry. I assured Arnie the man was in excellent health, and besides, while a bit unusual, this was actually a well-known technique. Arnie simply had to remain calm for it to work.

Later that day I got a call, not from the major, but from Arnie. To my amazement—and relief—he reported the intervention was successful. The major had marched bravely into the shop, Arnie was ready, dropped a snake around the man's neck, told him the snake's name was Molly, and wasn't she a lovely pet? The major froze, Arnie (bless him!) kept talking, and finally the major looked at the creature, realized he wasn't going to be attacked, and over the next hour, handled a number of Arnie's snakes. The next day, the major called, said he was fine, thanked me almost casually, and said he was looking forward to his deployment.

I tried the technique again in a similar situation, and it failed miserably. I never tried it again.

Unlike the major, most of my consultations were with officers seeking advice about problem people in their command. Typically, that might be someone who appeared to be depressed, or displayed some oddity of behavior.

About six weeks into my new position, a civilian with a badge of some sort asked if I would be willing to undertake some, well, call it "intelligence" work. It would involve being thoroughly vetted, of course, but my combination of medical and psychiatric training could be useful. I agreed—why not?—and was taken on a long walk around the corridors to a door guarded by two armed soldiers. That was strange enough, but the innocent-looking outer door turned out to be a cover for an inner door, an oval, metal door like one might see in a submarine movie. We stepped through that one into a narrow hallway jammed with electronic equipment and a line of tiny desks manned by a long row of people, busily turning knobs and looking at screens. I felt like I was suddenly in a submarine waiting for someone to yell, "DIVE!"

At this point, I have to inject a caution. When I was accepted into my new job, I signed a statement, DA Form 2962, saying I would "not divulge classified information orally, in writing, or by any other means." I took this to mean I would not *ever* divulge, etc., so I am being careful with this part of the narrative. What I am describing does not, in my view, intrude into any sacred realm.

We ended up in a small room with a "mirror" across the top of one wall, an obvious one-way window. This was to be a lie detector examination, so I was wired up and told we would talk a while before starting. I was read about ten or so questions to be asked during the test, we talked about them, then the test began. It was all pretty obvious stuff, no zingers, nothing Joseph McCarthy about any of it. However, the last question came out of the blue.

"Have you ever done anything illegal?"

When he asked, the image of doing abortions less than a year before popped into my head, and I simply said, "Yes."

That was it. Pending clearance from the FBI background check, I was hired. A few weeks later, my work for the Invisible Force began. Most of it was bland routine, focused principally on examining medical records for anything that could indicate substance abuse, use of "tranquillizers," sleeping drugs, or antidepressants, all thought to indicate possible instability, or vulnerability to manipulation. Anyone seen as overutilizing medical services was also suspect. It was all said to be cautionary, just being sure there wasn't something possibly sinister lurking in the background.

One issue that did make me uncomfortable, though, was the decidedly homophobic bias that came up frequently. At that time, the official psychiatric nomenclature described homosexuality as a personality disorder under the frightening rubric of Sociopathic Personality Disturbance, co-listed with Sexual Sadism and Pedophilia. In 1968, Sexual Deviation was given its own category, but Homosexuality was still grouped with Sadism and Pedophilia. In 1987, its designation as a disease was finally dropped.

There was nothing specific in the usual medical record to make one suspect homosexuality, nor did I worry that my personal objection to calling it a disease would clash with my duties. A few times my handler posed "theoretical" security situations to puzzle through, some involving a hint of homosexuality. In those situations, I chose my words carefully, staying right on the data path; that is, no speculation without solid evidence. My job, as I saw it, was to balance genuine security concerns with clarity and fairness.

One of my first consultations was with a colonel who ran a large personnel department, an innovative place where ideas to short-cut cumbersome procedures were evaluated. A large number of very bright career men and women were given relatively free rein to experiment with their ideas. This was a time when the emerging science of computers was being applied to solve some old problems.

The colonel had an embarrassing problem, the suspicion one of his assistants had allowed an unqualified person access to one of their most important evolving projects. The fox was in the henhouse and had to be extracted quickly. Could I look at the situation and manage a quick, quiet, by-the-book way out? It seems that an unexpected Specialist, or E-4, showed up with orders to begin work on a hush-hush project using a mysterious algorithm to prevent security threats from gaining entry into training programs.

An E-4 is an enlisted soldier with at least two years of service and training in a specific area, a rank just below sergeant. The man's orders were apparently unremarkable, and the clerk who processed him sent a hum-hum FYI note to someone further up the line approving his placement within the office. A few weeks into his placement, however, things started to go wrong. Oddly coded fragments, whose origin couldn't be traced, popped up randomly, at first just deleted and forgotten, but when they didn't stop, and in fact started to spell out bizarre ideas, the colonel was alerted. It was clear someone was messing with the system. Suspicion quickly fell on the newcomer, worry became alarm, and the colonel suspected he had a full-blown crisis on his hands. Would I please see the E-4 as soon as possible and advise if the colonel was right thinking the man had a mental disorder, and if so, what would be the next immediate step?

It didn't take long to find out the person involved was actually supposed to have been hospitalized at Walter Reed Hospital after being air evacuated from a hospital in Korea where he had been treated for Acute Paranoid Schizophrenia. This was one time the Army's usually flawless system of moving people around failed. The patient had been taken from the hospital to the air base, his records handed to him with a note on the front, "Walter Reed Hospital," to tell the triage people at Andrews AFB the correct bus for this particular patient. There was plenty of time on the long flight home to read the record and uncover all the malicious conclusions reached about his mental state and need for more care. Fortunately, being a personnel specialist, he knew exactly how to remedy the situation. He changed the triage note to "Pentagon," and when he got there, he went to the records department, asked for a clutch of blank forms, and before long had talked himself into the colonel's unit, sporting a pristine medical record, and vague hints about previous "special assignments" in security work.

When I saw the man, he was superficially cooperative, but it only took a few minutes for his bizarre plan for personnel improvements to unfold. I was amazed he had been able to pull off his delusional caper, but he did—almost. Arrangements were made on the spot to have him hospitalized, and the colonel returned to his unit to start repairing the damage.

I am not sure what happened to the patient, but with good care and supervision, his intelligence and verbal ability could well have resulted in a good outcome. Over the years, I have seen a large number of people with what seemed initially like impossible illness over time become highly successful in business and interpersonal relationships. Scant comfort for the colonel, but certainly true.

By the end of my first year as an almost-psychiatrist, it was clear to me I wanted to go further, especially since it also offered the chance for parallel study in neurology. The early psychiatrists evolved from neurology; in fact, the original term for the specialty was "Neuro-Psychiatrist." While the neurology part was falling away, one-third of the post-residency board certification examination was in neurology. You couldn't be board certified in psychiatry without knowing neurology.

There were a number of psychiatry residency programs in the area, so I shopped around, finally settling on a three-year residency at the Georgetown University Hospital. Ironically, one of its prior professors had been Harry Stack Sullivan, author of the interviewing book given to me by Colonel McGonagal on my first day as a psychiatrist. The program was heavily weighted toward the study of psychoanalysis, though I quickly realized that the Washington area was alive with influential psychiatric scholars, many open to alternatives to purely analytic/Freudian thinking. At first brush, the Georgetown program seemed non-doctrinaire about theories of human behavior—including biological theories that were starting to move in entirely new treatment directions. I over-read that part.

I was accepted, and at the same time, advised to start my own psychoanalysis, a rare opportunity to get started well ahead of the residency. While not a requirement of residency, it was still an expectation. If one later elected to go on into psychoanalytic training, after five years or so of "personal analysis," one could progress to a second or "training analysis." If not, one took the benefit of analysis into one's practice and personal life, a huge contribution to one's ability to practice effectively.

There was, of course, the little problem of being in the Army, having a full-time job that required rotating night and weekend duty, occasional field training, and wasn't inclined to give an inch on duty hours. The Georgetown Chief gave me several names, and I was lucky to find an analyst willing to work with my rigid schedule. We found a way for me to have four, fifty-minute, sessions a week. The price was $25.00 a session, and I had to agree that nothing would get in the way of a scheduled hour, that I would take my vacation when my analyst took his—traditionally in August—plus the tough part: I had to pay for the work out of pocket, no insurance or scholarships allowed. Earning the money was said to make the work more meaningful. Given my modest pay and the needs of my family, that meant I would have to get a second job—moonlighting.

Two of my Pentagon friends also needed extra money, so we formed a group, renting ourselves out to family practices for night and weekend coverage, rotating call every three days. A doctor's answering service was our go-between, taking patient information, then passing it and driving directions along to the on-call member. There were no cell phones or GPS systems, so once one was on the road, finding the destination depended entirely on the accuracy of the ladies at the answering service. Our fee was $10.00 for a basic visit, $15.00 if an injection was involved, cash or check. Typically, I would get from two to five calls between 6 p.m. and 6 a.m. when I went off duty.

We did that for a year. It paid for my analysis, sharpened my skills, the entire enterprise making subsequent life as a resident seem like a cake walk.

Of the many calls I received, the one that topped them all started with a warning, something like, "Look, Dr. Hirsh, I'm really sorry about this one, but they're gypsies. They said your patient is the King." We never refused a patient, so I set off having been warned not to expect payment. My directions took me to what appeared to be an abandoned house in Arlington, Virginia. I knocked (no doorbell) and was greeted by four or five men who eyed me suspiciously, and sure enough, seemed to be speaking Romani to each other. I was taken into the living room, an empty space without a stick of furniture, just blankets and quilts on the floor, a sort of community dormitory.

The patient was an elderly man, propped up against the wall, wrapped in a blanket. He didn't seem to notice me at all, but I could see from across the room the King was seriously ill. He was slumped over, sweating profusely, his breathing was labored, and he was severely dehydrated. More men gathered around, no women in sight, as I knelt to examine the man. It took all of two minutes to confirm he had pneumonia, the need for hospitalization both obvious and urgent. I told the group my findings, but they shook their heads in disagreement.

"You give him a shot," one said. It wasn't a suggestion; it was a command. I argued for a while, but it was obvious the old boy was going nowhere. They rejected the idea of a prescription for oral medication and repeated the demand I give him a magical injection. It was utterly useless to do otherwise, so I gave him a jolt of antibiotic, and prepared to leave. The group had stepped back to form a ring standing around the perimeter of the room. To my surprise, and contrary to what I had been led to expect, one of the group asked how much I was owed.

"Fifteen dollars," I said. He translated, the group seemed to find the fee acceptable, and he said I would be paid. He reached in his pocket, scratched about, came up empty handed, tried the other pockets without any luck, shrugged and said something to the man next to him. He went through his pockets. Nothing. And so it went, all the way around the circle of perhaps fifteen men. When it got back to the beginning, the spokesman said, "You send us a bill." I said I would and left for my next appointment. I hadn't gotten a dime, and sadly, I didn't give the King a chance of surviving another day.

Three days later, I got another call from the same house. Somehow, the old fellow was still alive, but there was very little life left in him. This time, the argument over hospitalization was brief,

I gave him a useless shot, and when the circle formed up, I said I'd send a bill and left. Two days later, there was an article in the paper saying that a gypsy king had died, and gypsies from a wide area were gathering. It was less a funeral notice than a warning to local merchants.

One of the other duties we all shared was night and weekend coverage. It was usually fairly quiet, but there were some atypical moments. One night, I was called to a bathroom where a cleaning lady was in the final stages of labor. I delivered the baby on the bathroom floor, and saw to their transport to a local hospital.

By far the most memorable night event involved a cousin I rarely got to see. He was in town for just one night, and I was on duty, so I suggested he come to the Pentagon. He was hesitant, but I convinced him we were easy to find, and our visit would be uneventful. He came, and while we were catching up, the phone rang, and the desk clerk told me a ranking officer was there and wanted to be seen immediately. I said I would be happy to see him, just give me a minute to get ready; meaning, give me time to get my cousin into another office.

"Sorry, sir, but he's already on his way." Almost instantly, there was a knock at the door. I didn't want to have to explain my cousin to a demanding officer, so I tossed a white coat to him, told him to put it on and be quiet. He didn't really have a choice.

The officer almost charged in, paid no attention to my introduction of—reading the name on the coat pocket—"Doctor Northworth," and immediately started talking about a highly personal problem. I was trapped. There was no way to stop him at that point, so I listened, and after what seemed like an eternity, I was asked for my advice. I gave it, he seemed satisfied, shook my hand and left. He didn't even seem to notice "Dr. Northworth." I had to face my cousin who by that point was apoplectic over the predicament I had thrust upon him. I apologized, but he left in a huff. I really can't blame him, though over time the incident was forgiven.

Another duty snag involved the Army's obsession with being in a constant state of readiness. Indeed, incessant training really did keep everything on the edge of action. That even included our pharmacy, and the plan the Army had to deal with it in case of war. Some genius came up with the idea that if the Pentagon came under attack, we should somehow manage to load all of the important medications into boxes, get a truck, and drive everything to Fort Meade, about an hour away in normal traffic, probably a little longer in a war.

All of it translated into actually practicing such a move. Every few months, on a Saturday morning, one of us had to supervise the entire process, starting (as usual) in the dark, and not finishing until well into the afternoon. The shelves were cleared, carefully packed into boxes, loaded into a truck, driven to Ft. Meade, then to a check point where an inspection would be done, and a precious confirmation signature obtained. Then the entire trip was reversed, the boxes were unloaded, and every bottle and tube placed back on the shelves in correct order. For whatever strange reason, the pharmacist was not part of the operation, but on Monday morning he had plenty to say if the drugs were not replaced exactly as they were on Friday night. It took six corpsmen, a truck, and a car to do the whole thing. Everyone hated it; happily, it happened so infrequently, most of us never had to do it. Maybe I would luck out.

Wrong. But even before my number came up, I had been thinking of ways to perhaps *streamline* the task, make it more efficient. After talking with the wise sergeant who ran the operation, it was clear the Ft. Meade turn around was just a formality. "Sometimes, when they're really busy, they don't even look in the truck. They just sign and tell us to get the hell out. That's why we go early, to get there before the crowd."

The solution seemed obvious: get the truck there when there *was* a crowd. Put a few drugs in a couple of boxes, cover up the empties with a big tarp, put a fat padlock on the truck door, leave at a civilized hour, like eight o'clock, get in line, make a to-do about getting the key to unlock the door, and hope they didn't do any more than glance in and sign the paper. I met with the men and told them if we did it this way, and everyone kept his mouth shut, I would buy breakfast, and the whole caper could be done before noon. If we got caught, I promised to take the heat. They agreed.

On Saturday, we loaded two boxes, staged the rest, had a nice breakfast on the road to Ft. Meade, timed our arrival to be in a line of trucks and cars, and when we got to the check point, the harried soldier wanted no part of our fumbling around for the key. He signed the paper, and we left. We returned the drugs, everyone pledged silence, and we all went home.

On Monday morning, I was told to report to the Colonel's office, *immediately*. Shit! How did he find out? No matter, I already had a cover story. How bad could it be?

When I got to the office, there was the Colonel, his adjunct, *and the pharmacist!* But weirdly, they were all smiling! Indeed, they were collectively delighted with the job we had done. The pharmacist was thrilled that we had returned all of the drugs to their rightful position.

"It's almost as if they were never moved."

The Colonel was so pleased, he said he was authorizing a new television to be put in the doctor's lounge. I said I thought it would be more appropriate in the enlisted men's lounge, "After all, they did all the work."

The television was installed, the men were happy, and I breathed a huge sigh of relief.

Protocol, practice, preparedness…it was all the glue that not only held everything together, but also made the Army so nimble. But sometimes, it seemed to go too far. Take the story of the not-dead dead general, for example. We got a call from a super-secure section of the building saying a four-star general had collapsed in the War Room, the sanctuary of sanctuaries. The team rushed off, our cardiologist in the lead. When they arrived, however, armed guards prevented them from entering. It was Catch-22: no one could enter the War Room without authorization, and no one but medical personnel could move the fallen officer. After some arguing, the cardiologist said he was in charge, thus authorized to authorize putting the general on the stretcher and bringing him out. By the time they worked it out and the general was extracted, he was dead. But the team dutifully performed full-on cardiac resuscitation all the way into the dispensary. When they lifted him onto a bed, the exercise in futility stopped. But the Colonel was horrified we had stopped and ordered the team to keep on.

"But, sir," the cardiologist said, "he's dead. Really dead."

"No," said the Colonel, "A general of his rank is not dead until the Surgeon General of his branch of service *says* he's dead. A helicopter has been sent to get him, so keep going until *he* says to stop."

Meanwhile, the man's wife had been picked up and brought to the dispensary, joining a gaggle of other officers gathering in the hallway. Every time the door opened, they could catch a glimpse of the frantic effort going on to save the patient. There was hope.

It took about a half hour for the SG (Surgeon General) to arrive. He strode in, took one look, said, "He's dead," and left. He broke the news to the man's wife, who leaped to her feet, rushed into the room, and threw herself on her husband's body. There was a tiny moment of silence before she recoiled, obviously horrified to feel the dead-awhile cool of his skin. She screamed and ran out of the room.

Protocol, it can be cruel.

Shortly after the dead general incident, I was injured on the job and taken to Walter Reed for surgery. During my convalescence, I was surrounded by soldiers recovering from grievous injuries suffered in Vietnam. My own situation seemed shamefully trivial compared to the agony those men were experiencing. I knew firsthand the pain faced by soldiers with mental illness, but I hadn't seen physical injuries up close, or watched the inch by miserable inch fight for recovery. It's one thing to see war in a newsreel or movie where winning the battle is everything, patriotic pride is stirred, and the wounded are shuffled off for treatment with everyone's prayers and wishes for a speedy recovery. It's quite another when you hear their groans at night or watch as they struggle through family visits trying to mask their distress.

A few weeks before I left the Army, my intelligence handler came to me with a problem, this one right in our own unit. It had come to his attention that one of our men had been seen coming out of a bar said to cater to "homosexuals." I put that word in quotes not just because the uncomfortable anachronism was the accepted word used at the time, but more to the point: one larded with contempt in its many forms.

This was an awful situation. The man was not only loved by everyone in the unit, he was also approaching retirement after thirty years of flawless work. If the suspicion was "founded," he would not only be summarily discharged but lose all of his retirement benefits. It was a black and white situation. No wiggle room.

I suggested that given the enormity of the situation, I couldn't possibly draw any conclusions without interviewing the man to properly evaluate the situation. I dragged it out as much as possible, thinking there might be some way around it, but there wasn't, so I saw him and spelled out what I knew. He acknowledged being gay, and was, of course, devastated. The visit to the bar was the first and only time he had been there. After we talked a while, it was clear he had scrupulously monitored his behavior over the years. There was no evidence he was gay except the observation of some anonymous snoop whose report alone could destroy the man's life.

We talked a while, and I finally "realized" he had actually gone into the bar to help another soldier he worried might be headed down an evil path. It was a brave act to save a comrade. I reported my findings to a very skeptical handler. But he had said my report would carry the day, and so that was the end of it. It was also the end of my career in intelligence. I was removed from service, reminded of my obligation under Form 2962, and prepared to leave the Army.

A few days before I left, I spent the day doing exit physical exams for people leaving the Service. They were all unremarkable except one, a young corporal from another unit, someone I had never met before. She was accompanied by a nurse from her unit, odd because our own nurses usually chaperoned when we examined a female patient.

This time, however, there was something else going on. I could feel it. The corporal was obviously quite nervous, and the nurse was cold and irritable with her. It was as if the girl had done something terribly wrong, and boy! was she going get it from the doctor. Her history was unremarkable, and nothing showed up in the physical—until the pelvic examination. She was pregnant. It was early, her uterus only slightly enlarged, but it was then clear what all the *sturm und drang* was about.

I didn't allow my expression to change, went about it deliberately, and when I finished, I said to the girl. "Everything looks good. I wish you luck." The nurse was smoldering, and between clenched teeth said, "Are you absolutely sure...*Doctor?*" I said I was, signed the report, and opened the office door. The nurse went out first, and as the corporal left, she turned her head and mouthed a silent, "Thank you."

It was definitely time for me to leave. I went through several check-out stations, the last one dealing with any leave time not taken over the past two years, and thus owed as extra pay. The gay sergeant was at that desk.

"Well, Captain, I think there's been a mix-up in your record."

"Here we go again," I thought.

"It says you used fifty-six of your sixty leave days, but I think it's the other way around. It seems to me you only took four days. We owe you for the other fifty-six."

And that was the end of my two years in the United States Army. I can't close this chapter, however, without saying how much being in the Army meant to me. I saw a world I had never before imagined, played a microscopic part in one of our country's most controversial missions, and was challenged in ways inconceivable in civilian life. In spite of its astounding complexity, the Army ran efficiently and, above all, with *honor*. My respect for the Army, in spite of the era-based issues I mentioned, was and remains profound.

Everyone could benefit from exposure to military training. But the days of the draft ended almost fifty years ago, and only the most motivated volunteer steps up today. The rest aren't remotely interested. The medical corps has shrunk to about 4,400 career physicians on active duty, while at the same time, veteran's medical services have exploded. There are now roughly nine million veterans, a significant portion being cared for through the VA health system. That system has 1,243 health care facilities, 170 hospitals, and over a thousand out-patient sites. The VA employs over 11,000 physicians, though because of budgetary restrictions and frequent turnover, the GAO (Government Accountability Office) is unable to say exactly how many are full time, part time, in residency programs, or outside physician consultants. I'll have more to say later about this vital part of the nation's health care system.

I left the Pentagon on a Wednesday afternoon, this time not pressed for time or anxious about starting residency the next day. The Fates couldn't resist throwing in a little irony: my first placement was the in-patient psychiatric service at the VA hospital in Washington, DC. Same job, different uniform.

6

RESIDENCY
ALMOST THERE

OF ALL MY TRAINING EXPERIENCES, the one I would most willingly swap for today's model would be psychiatric residency. My motivation and expectations would be the same now as then: to combine medical training with an understanding of behavior in order to be able to separate emotional issues from organic (physical) disorders, and know how best to treat each. But my mistake in 1967 was underestimating the control of the profession by psychoanalytic forces.

While I understood the vital role of personal analysis, and respected historical analytic theory, I thought the emergence of better medication, coupled with gains in brain chemistry and genetic research, were putting the specialty on the brink of an entirely new approach to mental illness. Thorazine started the tectonic shift, and I thought the plates were on the move again. I saw a changing specialty, and I wanted to be part of it.

Strangely, I would not have made the swap as recently as ten years ago. At that point, psychiatry seemed doomed to become a medication-dependent, assembly-line specialty headed for oblivion. In 2010, residencies were only about one-third full, adding a mere 483 graduates to the 28,000 psychiatrists in the US that year. More were dying off or retiring than entering the field. It seemed like a hopeless situation.

But suddenly, things changed. Now residencies are 97% filled, highly competitive, and the number of graduates has doubled. Why the abrupt turnaround? The short answer is: *Awareness, Science,* and *Compensation.*

Awareness: Word has finally filtered down that the analyst's couch has been sent to Goodwill, replaced by research-based, outcome-focused care delivered on multiple levels. At the same time, the public has been alerted by the crushing tragedy of teenage suicide, now ranking the third most common cause of death between 12 and 19, the opioid crisis, school and church shootings, woeful lack of mental health screening services, and the realization that most homeless people, especially Veterans, and a disproportionate number of incarcerated persons, are not simply ne'er-do-wells and criminals, but people with mental illness brushed off the board by indifference and lack of more appropriate treatment options.

Demand for substance abuse treatment opportunities has increased dramatically as the stigma associated with seeking mental health care in general has fallen. Primary care physicians, the courts, schools, and prison officials have all been increasingly vocal in their frustration with the lack of available care. The list goes on.

People at every level are changing their understanding of mental illness, moving from accepting the need for change to *demanding* it. In 2010, psychiatry ranked 9th in the number of people searching for referral. It is now 2nd, just behind the number looking for primary care appointments.

Science. Research in brain function and a host of related issues are not only advancing but have moved from theoretical to practical, information practitioners use every day in patient care. Patients, too, expect scientific explanations of their problems and treatment. Jokes about blaming a behavior on childhood mishap have been replaced by serious discussions of the lasting effect of real childhood trauma. Witness the dramatic explosion in exposing and dealing effectively with sexual trauma. Once crushed under the weight of shame and anger, the demon is now on the run.

Similarly, look at the emerging understanding of the complexity of Substance Abuse, helped at the same time by pressure on insurers to cover SA services. Not long ago, inpatient programs were limited, and both inpatient and outpatient work were largely under the purview of Alcoholics Anonymous (AA). As effective as AA is, it is not science based, and its appeal and demands do not suit all sufferers. Today, AA group principles are alive and well, especially in aftercare, but medication and cognitive and other therapies have vastly increased the scope and effectiveness of treatment.

Denial of SA treatment in prison has been one of the cruelest and most shortsighted aspects of "punishment." Indeed, the entire issue of punishment is suddenly under review. Attention has turned to more sensible sentencing guidelines, effective mental illness diagnosis and treatment, restoration justice, job training, and post-incarceration programs. Punishment is still there, but on the most practical level, it is now clear that a rational overhaul of the system salvages lives, along with reaping huge financial dividends.

A decade ago, few medical students were drawn to a specialty whose only function seemed to be dispensing a small group of drugs to people in dead-end situations. But dramatic changes in perception and teaching have produced an enormous increase interest in psychiatry as a career.

Compensation. Resident salaries in the mid-1960s averaged $3,000–$6,000 a year. Today, across all specialties, residents average $55,000–$70,000. In the past, those of us just coming out of service could qualify for a $3,600-a-year training stipend. With some personal savings added in, it was just enough for me to stop moonlighting, continue analysis four times a week, and live a modest but comfortable resident's life.

In practice settings, Public Health, Pediatrics, Family Practice, and Psychiatry have always been the least lucrative specialties. Pediatricians, by the way, are a special breed, always among the most dedicated of all physicians, far more passionate about their patients than about money. The same motivation has long been a large part of public health service and family medicine. While their position on the money scale is largely unchanged, better paying jobs, aggregation in more efficient practice settings, and thaws in insurance reimbursement have boosted the group from the basement to the first floor.

The bottom line is that psychiatry is finally fusing with mainstream medicine. Residencies are offering robust training, research continues to highlight new treatments, and the public is shaking off some of the stigma that has poisoned the well for so long. In every aspect of health care delivery, there are ongoing insurance, political, and Pharma-greed battles still to be fought, but the issues are now out in the open for all to see and debate.

There is yet another reason to make the swap: today's comprehensive training does a vastly better job of preparing emerging psychiatrists for specialty board examinations, typically given after two years in practice. In the mid-1960s, the boards were almost an afterthought, and many psychiatrists chose to skip them entirely.

The "Boards" are not mandatory; unlike the lawyer's Bar exam, you don't need them to be licensed to practice. By that point in one's career, licensing issues have all been settled by the prior national and some state exams. The amount of time and resources needed to prepare make boards an extension of the residency, a test focused only on one's specialty, the first of a series of continuing education courses and tests reaching into the distance.

The first-attempt pass rate for all the boards varies from 70–90%. Exams are given yearly, and can be repeated. They're also expensive. To continue one's state medical license, physicians have long been required to document 30–50 hours of study in certified CME programs every year. In 1990, the specialty boards jumped on the bandwagon, demanding a ten-hour recertification examination every ten years on top of the state requirements.

About 85% of physicians are board certified, but for a number of reasons, many choose not to take the test at all. Some see it

as a money-making enterprise designed to advance the business model of medical care. They point out the fact that board
certified physicians can command higher wages simply because
of a test result, not because they necessarily have greater skill
levels compared to their colleagues. Others feel at a disadvantage because they practice within a narrowly defined branch of
their specialty. To prepare means taking an enormous amount
of time to show minute knowledge outside their specialty range.
Some feel the tests are nothing more than a vanity issue, not an
objective measure of skill.

The problem with psychiatry boards when I trained was that
the boards were comprehensive, and our training was not—starting with a lack of attention to neurology. The exams were given
in two parts, starting with two days of written tests, followed
a year later by two days of oral examinations. One third of the
four-day examination was on neurology, yet as I discovered to my
dismay, neurology was hardly mentioned during residency. What
was *not* emphasized on the board exams was therapy—analytic
or otherwise. The boards tested knowledge across the entire field:
brain chemistry, public health, statistics, substance abuse, plus
everything imaginable about medications. Freud and Jung? No.
Neurochemistry? Yes.

As a result, I spent a considerable amount of my first year in
practice relearning neurology, then another year reviewing basic
science. By the time I took the exam, I was dead certain I knew
the subject, and actually enjoyed the experience, especially the
two days of oral examination.

But on that long-ago first day of residency, boards were the
last thing on my mind. I joined nine colleagues, including two
women, to start the last three years before we could begin practice. The entire first year—then as now—was devoted to inpatient
work with a supportive didactic program focused almost entirely
on diagnosis and medication treatment. Every Saturday morning, we gathered at a professor's house for literature and journal
review. Standard stuff.

My first assignment was at the Veteran's Hospital in Washington, DC, an enormous, up-to-speed facility with an inpatient psychiatric patient population of about 60 patients living Army-style in wards of twenty patients each. With residents on each ward, and two full-time attending psychiatrists supervising our work, we were in an ideal learning situation. My time at Chambers Pavilion was frontier medicine compared to the VA hospital, though there was a lot to be said for the intense "Do One" quality of learning in San Antonio.

The patients were a varied lot, some acutely ill transfers from active-duty service hospitals, but mostly veterans with recurring illness. Here's where it got tricky. The vast majority of patients with recurring or treatment resistant disorders received disability payments from the VA—not Social Security—the amount measured as a percentage of base pay. The percentage system was the same across all medical, surgical, and psychiatric categories of illness. For example, a mild form of depression, intrusive and inhibiting but not devastating, might be rated as 10%–30%, whereas more disruptive problems could go to 100%. If that veteran also had recurring gout rated at 10%, and hearing loss from battlefield noise rated at 30%, the total disability payment each month would be 140% of base pay. If a veteran had just a 40% rating but was admitted for inpatient care, the payment went up to 100% for the entire time of hospitalization, often complicating our ability to move patients through efficiently.

All of these financial intricacies were well known by our patients. Some didn't care, they just wanted to get well and leave. Many came as direct referral from outpatient clinics, but quite a few were veterans with chronic illness, men and women struggling to stay on their feet outside the hospital but ultimately dependent on the VA system both medically and financially. Many of those veterans were probably suffering from unacknowledged PTSD, a diagnosis yet to break into our awareness.

Finally, there were some who, quite frankly, milked the system. Among that group were some who traveled between VA hospitals on a regular basis. In the winter, they went south; in the summer, they came back north. The most egregious of the lot was one patient who arrived (again) carrying his suitcase in one hand, and a bowling ball in a custom leather case in the other.

It gets trickier. The line between manipulation and the real deal was not always easy to see. VA hospitals talked with each other in an effort to control the abuse issue, but when there was a question, the veteran always received the benefit of doubt. Also, pressure for discharge often produced acting out behavior, sometimes a reflection of the severity of the underlying disorder, sometimes a conscious manipulation. I saw both in my time at Chambers Pavilion.

Getting patients to accept discharge was a major part of our everyday work. To get an idea of how ready a patient was, we encouraged a pass away from the hospital. It could be a day, several days or a week, each part of the continuum leading to discharge. Even so, we sometimes got it wrong, most frequently when a patient left on pass and disappeared, often reappearing at another VA hospital seeking admission. But it could also be worse than that. One of our patients committed suicide on pass, something none of us saw coming. Even in the exhaustive review, there did not appear to be any clear warning signs, underlining the fact that not all suicide is predictable or even a function of depression. Anger, intense feelings of rejection, hypersensitivity to perceived injury in severely narcissistic people, fear of protracted illness… the list is long.

Talking about manipulative patients and disability harvesting is as risky, and it is necessary. The hazard is appearing judgmental, or even dismissive of certain patients. In anticipation of that sentiment, keep in mind that such behavior is a fact of life everywhere—in all medical environments. Also, remember these cases are the exception, not the rule. Nor are they benign. They are disruptive, time consuming, expensive, and too often perilous.

The spectrum of disability gaming runs from pure, lazy manipulation to acts of desperation driven by a host of issues, most commonly poverty and inability to sustain even minimal employment. Substance abuse lies behind a disturbing number of cases. Some imagine an easy way to subsidize a passive lifestyle; others are hopelessly trapped in abuse, and disability offers a desperate way to hang on.

In both the VA and civilian world, the application process for any medical or psychological illness is the same: if you are disabled, unable to work for a year, and have not improved with repeated treatment, you can apply for disability income. In the civilian world, application is through one of two Social Security programs: either SSI or SSDI. SSDI is for people who have been employed, paid sufficiently into Social Security to be "insured," thus entitled to benefits. SSI is a special needs program for those not sufficiently invested to get full benefits. To qualify, the recipient's assets are carefully evaluated ("means tested"). By the current rules, you can own a car, but otherwise not have a net worth of more than $2,000.

Application for either follows a predictable path, starting with the near certainty of rejection of the first application, often absurdly so—as if an orangutan with a rejection stamp was the only employee in the First Time Department. A nurse I once worked with in a mental health clinic was overtaken by brain cancer, bedridden at home when she applied, and in a coma when she was rejected.

The same thing happens with the second try. Additional letters, clinical reports, and lab work are gathered, and again, it is likely to be rejected. Around that time, patients turn to disability lawyers. They won't take a case until it has been rejected two or three times, then they step in, challenge the rejections, and through persistence, eventually win a hearing. Witnesses are called, arguments are made, the system is worn down, most of the time, resulting in approval. At that point, the question turns to the fuzzy issue of exactly when the disability began, important because there are two payments to consider: back pay and monthly allowance. The monthly part is pretty easy, but saying exactly when it all started is harder. Once the argument is settled and a date set, the back pay sum is calculated by multiplying the number of months times the monthly allowance. The lawyer keeps that part for his trouble.

There is a certain type of depression associated with disability, one with a paradoxical onset following a successful review. Elation over winning quickly gives way to the realization that victory means continuation of poverty. Furthermore, if you are able to do some work to supplement your income, but not enough to support yourself and surrender your disability income, you have to be sure not to earn more than $880 a month, or your benefits will be challenged. Of course, Social Security wants you to return to the work force, and many do. But for those who need to stay on disability and still earn some money, the underground economy often becomes the answer.

Disability benefits include Medicare (SSDI) and Medicaid (SSI), though there are catches, starting with a two-year waiting period for Medicare—and it is not free. Its premiums and copays can eat up a sizeable part of one's monthly benefits. Medicaid starts immediately, is free, though means tested, and its rules vary by state, some more restrictive than others.

My point in going into detail about such a seemingly arcane subject is to highlight a really difficult part of a physician's job across all specialties, starting with helping people avoid the need for disability in the first place, as well as filtering out those who are trying to game the system. Next, there is the daunting task of helping patients cope with the limits of disability, while simultaneously encouraging movement toward autonomy, both physical and financial.

"Disability" has also become entangled in political discussion, often quite polarizing. SSDI payments are classed as "entitlements," taking roughly 4% of the federal budget. For many, the very word "entitlement" triggers the same salivary response as "welfare," and any well-publicized case of fraud underscores the righteousness of condemnation.

But the exception does not prove the rule.

Still, there is no question about the enormous cost to taxpayers, something that has triggered many legislative attempts to control cost while preserving the core idea of helping the disabled. Sometimes regulatory constriction produces a huge backlash, followed by compensatory retreat. I remember one vivid example of a proposal to review all disability recipients with an eye on eliminating any undeserved payments. Letters announcing the plan caused panic. The legalese was both hard to interpret and menacing, but the message was clear: if you can show you really are disabled, you have nothing to fear. It was hardly a comfort to people with no idea if or when the hammer could fall, or how they were going to prove their case. The backlash was instant, the threat was reversed, but fear lingered that it would happen again.

Beyond cost, some critics point to fluctuations in application rates as evidence of abuse. When the economy is good, rates fall, and when there is a downturn, applications increase. It's tempting to conclude that disability has to be a padded phenomenon: when things go bad, people look for the government to help out. The truth is more nuanced. We are largely talking about people who live on the margin, so a good economy means more jobs, closer to home, and more accommodating than when jobs are scarce. A faltering economy means employers can pick from a larger pool with fewer issues. Applying for disability becomes the only option.

My experience over the past fifty years in hospitals, private practice, and public health clinics gives me a huge patient base from which to draw my conclusions, starting with the fact that most disabled people are exactly that: disabled. Even partial disability can be crippling when it comes to earning a living. Yes, there are those who game the system, but they are few in number—perhaps 1–2%. And what do they get for their effort? Better put: what is the average support disabled persons receive? Peanuts. Can you imagine living on $6,000–$12,000 a year, with Medicare premiums on top of that? How hard would you fight to capture that flag? Images of a "welfare queen" behind the wheel of a Cadillac, or tales of people pretending all manner of physical illness while living in a beachfront condo, are somewhere between extreme rarity and pure propaganda.

Dr. Martin Luther King was assassinated in April 1968 just as I was preparing to move to my next assignment. Four days later, a large part of the nation's capital went up in flames. I watched from the roof of the VA hospital.

My next inpatient assignment was at the District's only public hospital, DC General Hospital, a sprawling complex serving the city's poorest residents, a wild zoo of a place where every imaginable illness, accident, and category of mental difficulty circulated at any given moment—as far from the homogenized VA as it is possible to imagine. It opened in 1806 and closed in 2011 when the city was facing bankruptcy. It's funny how easy it is to cut services to the most vulnerable in times of fiscal stress.

The psychiatric part consisted of an outpatient clinic with 24-hour emergency services covering one-half of all of the District of Columbia, and a modest inpatient unit housing four patients to a room, a few offices, and a large day room. That was it. Get 'em in, get 'em out. Unlike the VA, no one wanted to linger on the inpatient service, especially in the summer when temperatures were sweltering. And why was there no air conditioning? Catch-22 in full bloom.

Under DC's bureaucratic system, qualifying for AC started with documentation of need. Easy enough, you say: just record the temperature four times a day for a week or two, send it in, plug in the units. Simple, right? No. The rules say you have to document over multiple months extending well into the fall to prove your case. Only then you can submit your request. Okay, a delay, maybe, but then you'll have relief next summer, right? Nope, wrong again. Two months isn't long enough to get anyone's attention, and after the first of the new year, no old requests could be considered. Sorry, you'll have to start the process over again next summer. So, there was no AC.

The patient population was varied but always on the wild side, especially when we had hallucinating alcoholics in withdrawal, rejected for care on medical wards. Or agitated schizophrenic patients, wound up manic patients, or "Borderlines" whose behavioral specialty was both cutting and suicide attempts—the latter always a surprise and potentially lethal. Many of our patients wouldn't dream of taking medication or cooperating with staff, much less attend follow-up appointments. It was a challenging place to work, cramped, stifling in any season, and because we did not lock doors, a constant threat a patient would simply walk out and disappear.

The nursing staff was chronically overwhelmed, and suicide attempts were a frequent occurrence, some quite bizarre. One desperate man broke several razor blades into small pieces, swallowed the lot, and went to bed expecting to quietly bleed out in the night. When he woke up in the morning, he was so disappointed he told us what he had done. Fortunately, the body has a defense against sharp objects passing through the gut (coats them in thick mucus), and except for some unpleasant nicks around the aft portal, he was all right. We believed him when he said he wouldn't ever do that again.

Patients usually brought their few belongings in a battered suitcase, laundry sack, or a cardboard box, all of it stored under their bed—no bureaus or closets in this hospital. Making rounds one night, the nurse noticed a sleeping man's arm hanging down, his hand in the box of clothes just under the edge of his bed. Nothing unusual. In the morning, he was found dead from loss of blood from a deeply lacerated wrist. He had waited until all was quiet, cut his arm, dangled it just out of sight in the box, and passed out. The clothing and box soaked up the blood, so it didn't leak out on the floor where it could be seen.

The outpatient part of our service saw every sort of case, including children. By far the most amazing of those was a boy of eight who came for regular outpatient treatment, the object of concern and amazement to all of us. He was largely mute, rarely saying anything beyond a few random words. He was close to pleasant, flat without seeming to be despondent, cooperative when pressed, but clearly living in his own internal world, one that only occasionally took note of outside events. Ninety-five percent of his time was spent drawing cereal boxes from memory, exact replicas of any of a dozen brands like Corn Flakes, Raisin Bran, and the rest. His drawings were perfect in every tiny detail, down to the patent numbers and list of contents, each spelled out in dead-straight lines, each letter and number an uncanny reproduction of the original.

There was some debate about diagnosis, but it came down to either childhood schizophrenia or what in those days was called, "*Idiot Savant.*" Today, the diagnosis would likely be an Autism Spectrum variant, somewhere between autism and Asperger's Disorder, both officially recognized in 1980. The boy's fluid movements and mutism favor the Autism side, his prodigious memory more characteristic of Asperger's. It's entirely speculative, and whatever the diagnosis, it was an amazing experience to spend time with this fellow, watch him work so effortlessly, simultaneously unaware or simply uninterested in whatever was going on around him.

I saw several others with the Idiot Savant label during training, most memorably, a fellow who had memorized the entire Philadelphia transportation system. Give him a starting point, time, and destination, and he would instantly reel off what bus to take, when, where, and how to transfer—the entire trip in rapid fire sequence.

A substantial number of our referrals came to us in handcuffs, people the police either knew to be mentally ill or thought they might be. The rules for informed consent were pretty lax, and we were expected to take whoever came our way so the cops could get back to work. One night around midnight, they brought in a young man, well-dressed, fairly calm, coherent, and reluctant to discuss his situation in front of the police. He had been caught standing on the outside edge of a bridge fifty feet above a busy parkway, apparently just about to leap.

He denied being depressed, but who jumps off a bridge if he isn't depressed or completely around the bend? Wrong affect again, so sensing we were going nowhere, I told the cops we would hospitalize the man, they left, and I asked what was *really* going on. After a few anxious minutes, he confessed the truth: "I was taking a leak. I couldn't just piss in the street, so I climbed over the rail where I didn't think anyone would see me." After a brief discussion of what a bad idea that was, we called him a cab and sent him on his way.

Not all cases that didn't add up were as easily solved, but like Mr. James getting run over by spies in San Antonio, or the more benign tale of the man who just looked like he was about to jump off the bridge, the moral of the story is always the same: stick with the basics—don't get distracted by appearances.

Take the bizarre care of Edna Hilevich. It started with a routine request from the main ER on the other side of the hospital campus. A disheveled, incoherent woman with no ID was brought in by police, apprehended on the sidewalk in front of a movie theater, screaming at the ticket taker. Obviously, a nut case, the police reasoned, so let DC General figure it out, starting with the main ER to be sure she didn't have a medical problem. The cops didn't want to take any chances: they had been burned too many times mistaking diabetics in metabolic trouble for people with mental illness. A neurologist was called, but the patient was far too agitated for a decent examination. They got some blood—no answers there—and felt it unlikely she was having some kind of stroke variant. Then they called us. I did my best to talk to her, but she seemed to ignore me, gesturing and yelling in an unrecognizable language. Thorazine had the same effect on her as it did Mr. James: it slowed her down a bit, but nothing else changed. Strange. Nothing fits.

We transported her to the unit, did our best to help her calm down, cleared a room just for her, and had our most experienced nurse stay with her until exhaustion and Thorazine finally knocked her out. It was the same the next morning, but by then we started to think there was more to her rant than pure psychosis. Maybe she's deaf, we thought. We tried to startle her with sudden noise behind her back, but it was inconclusive. I begged the ENT resident to see her on our unit since taking her to him in the main hospital was way out of the question. His conclusion: she was almost completely deaf. He rigged some sort of amplifier, put the bud in her ear, and for the first time since she arrived, she stopped yelling; well, sort of stopped, at least briefly. She started to talk to the resident, loudly, but not screaming. Also, her voice, tone and rapidity of speech changed, suggesting that being able to hear something allowed better phonation. It didn't take too long before a laundry worker identified her language as Polish.

Translating as best she could, the laundress said her name was Edna Hilevich, and she was agitated because her home had been destroyed. Using the police report to pinpoint the location of the theater, one of the nurses went there, took a Polaroid photo, and when Edna saw it, the story finally started to make sense. Edna grew up in a house long ago demolished to make way for the theater. She left the States at age five to live in Poland. For reasons I don't recall, she had come back to the states and tried to find her childhood home. It was gone! Someone had destroyed her home!

Over the next few days, Edna was able to calm down, Social Services located temporary housing with a Polish family while they continued to try to reconnect her with family, the ENT resident made follow-up arrangements, and we said a fond goodbye to Edna Hilevich.

Once again, the lesson was clear: an atypical, dramatic presentation makes it too easy to overlook an alternative explanation, label the patient, and push her off for someone else to deal with.

At the end of the year, I left DC General to start the next twelve months divided between child psychiatry and intensive instruction in psychotherapy—individual, group, and toward the end of the year, Family Therapy, then an emerging, still-controversial subspecialty. Along with inpatient work, the first year had focused heavily on interview technique and diagnosis, coincident with the publication of *DSM-II* in 1968, the first update of the original manual of psychiatric diagnosis since 1952. It was fairly anemic but at least took a shot at stabilizing diagnostic criteria, twelve years ahead of *DSM-III,* the first really comprehensive attempt to define and classify diagnosis using proven scientific studies.

What was entirely missing from our first year was any mention of neurology. Along with inpatient experience, today's residents are taught an integrated program of psychiatry and neurology right from the start. They are also exposed from the beginning to all forms of treatment, not just medication management. The list includes the intricacies of medication effects and mishaps, ECT and other forms of brain stimulation, child psychiatry, hospice programs, forensics, brain injury, PTSD, geriatric psychiatry, and extensive training in understanding and treating substance disorders.

One residency director told me the surprising fact that a small number of residents not only undertake personal analysis but continue into analytic training. Today, roughly 3,000 of the county's 28,000 psychiatrists are analysts; over thirty analytic training programs are still active. The numbers are deceptive, however, because most practitioners are older, average age in the upper 60s. More to the point, virtually none have a full-time analytic practice; in fact, they average between one and three patients, less because of interest than cost. Insurance won't go near analysis, and the out-of-pocket cost—up to hundreds of dollars per hour three to four times a week—is highly selective.

There still remains an active interest in learning dynamic and interpersonal theories rooted in analytic principles. That said, the majority of residents will go into "biological work," code for "medication management." Maximum medication, minimum conversation. As the same dean put it, "It's all about health care economics. Our graduates are no different from physicians joining any other specialty—they go where the money is."

One subspecialty area that has remained fundamentally unchanged is "Liaison Psychiatry," hospital-based consultation between referring physician and a psychiatrist dealing with any of a wide range of concerns, including assessing capacity to give informed consent, managing a known psychiatric problem in a medical or surgical setting, assessing self-harm risk, distinguishing delirium (short-term, reversible cognitive disruption) from dementia (multiple types of cognitive decline, generally progressive), diagnosing a suspected contiguous or "comorbid" condition, and to me the most intriguing of all: figuring out to what degree emotional issues—conscious or otherwise—are causing or complicating diagnostic and treatment problems. Beyond giving patients answers to thorny questions, it also shortens hospital stays and saves money.

A good example of a liaison would be resolving the complex question of how to use psychiatric medication in a Parkinson 's disease patient who develops psychotic symptoms. It is particularly tricky because the area of the brain responsible for Parkinson's symptoms is also exquisitely sensitive to the side effects of drugs used to control psychosis. Here, collaboration is the key to improvement.

Requests coming from the surgical service often involve sudden post-operative changes in behavior, ranging from an aberrant reaction to anesthesia to the abrupt onset of psychosis for no apparent reason. Hallucinations two to three days following surgery can reveal an unacknowledged addiction to alcohol—Delirium Tremens, or "DTs." While heroin addiction is too obvious to miss from the start, in recent times, complications from opioid addiction have tragically become more frequent than life-threatening issues with alcohol.

My first liaison consultation was easily the most memorable. A young woman, admitted for routine surgery, was found to have an overwhelming form of an untreatable cancer. In just two hours, she went from a healthy, vibrant graduate student with a career in epidemiology at her fingertips to a shattered soul with only a few months to live. Her reaction was as you might expect: horror, disbelief...and rage. Kubler-Ross' seminal book *On Death and Dying*, with its insights about the stages of dying from denial to acceptance, appeared a year later. Even if I had had it in hand, it would not have helped in the immediate moments I first met the patient.

As you might expect, she was furious over the suggestion she talk to a psychiatrist, especially a *resident* psychiatrist. She had been equally vigorous in her rejection of any pastoral help. She had thrown her family out of her room when they told her she simply had to accept the help of a priest. When I arrived, the family was in the hallway crying and arguing. The doctor was unsure what would happen when he introduced me, but we went in together, he left, and Cynthia simply stared at me. I told her I knew about her condition, her rejection of the priest, and the probability she would feel the same about me.

After a long minute, she said with calm sarcasm, "And exactly what do you propose to do to help me? Take away the cancer? Send me home to get back to work on my thesis?"

I told her I didn't have any answers at all, and I thought she had every right to react as she had. If that included throwing me out, it would be totally understandable. I told her I knew about the bleak and certain outcome but thought there could be other ways to gain at least a modicum of control over the situation.

That was the start of a three-month process continuing from her discharge up to the time she had to be admitted for the last time. But in those weeks, I worked with a remarkable woman who found her way through hopelessness to accept what was happening to her, starting from the chaotic moment her physician first told her about the cancer. There was a medical student with the surgeon when he broke the news, but the student became so overwrought, he left the room. That fueled her rage as much as the diagnosis itself. We worked from there.

The medical student was not criticized for his reaction because the situation was beyond anything he had previously been taught. With the help of my supervising psychiatrist, I looked into the medical school curriculum and found there was no attempt at any point in any discipline—including psychiatry—to help medical students deal with death and dying.

Kubler-Ross applied that observation in a far more generalized way, noting a societal lack of courage in dealing with the most thunderously inevitable fact of being: we are all going to die. *How we die is the question.*

Cynthia dealt with the idea of being dead with surprising dispatch. She had no concern about an afterlife, a fact that continued to get in the way of rapprochement with her family. To her, the burning issue was the terrible sense she would die without having accomplished anything significant or lasting. Putting that together with the grievous absence of teaching anything about dying, we talked about the idea of filming her as she went through the process, talking about herself, her diagnosis, and her painful path toward death. Used as a teaching tool for medical students, her accomplishment would be both courageous and lasting. Who would imagine that *adding* pain to the process could be her gift to naïve, invisible students? But she did it, and as the weeks passed, increasing weakness only made her more determined to see it through as far as she could.

Even when she finally reached the point of collapse, she thanked us for giving her a sense of purpose in those awful weeks. She was admitted and died within hours. And, yes, her family was there, and did respect her wish not to be attended by clergy.

The department was squeamish about the film, especially when they heard Cynthia dismiss concern for her soul's destiny, or her rejection of prayer as a possible way to alter the course of her illness. Being a Catholic hospital, the film would need approval by mysterious higher-ups.

The suggestion came back that if the offending parts were edited out, it might be approved. I argued that would be an unacceptable betrayal of Cynthia's trust.

At that point, the tape simply disappeared and was never mentioned again. I continued to use her story in teaching situations and will always be awed by her accomplishment.

The issue of religion was a delicate matter best avoided, but when it did surface, one had to tiptoe around it carefully. One of my greatest disappointments was the cowardice of the core of analytic teachers who refused to bring religion into the same arena as any other important life force demanding careful examination. Analysts in the program were all rigidly doctrinaire about the rules of analysis, insisting that nothing, absolutely nothing, was off the table. Except religion. As many times as I challenged the idea, or cited Freud and other luminaries on the subject, the response was always the same: out of bounds. Jewish analysts working for the department were more willing to talk about it openly, but even so, the attitude was, "Well, you know how it is, and when you're on your own, you can follow your instincts."

In the meantime, minus one topic, everything we were taught was modeled on psychoanalytic theory, starting with intensive analytically oriented psychotherapy, variously called "insight therapy," "psychodynamic therapy," or simply "dynamic therapy." The word "dynamic" is misleading. It usually means energetic, animated, or zestful, but in psychiatry it describes a *process*, a constantly *evolving system*. The business of therapy is to explore that system. Thus, therapy becomes an intensive collaboration between doctor and patient to find and weigh the causal progression of elements in the patient's life, and how those forces shaped the patient's personality, thinking, and problems. From there, the patient can assume command of previously unconsciously-driven, counter-productive behavior, a process called, "working through," as in practicing what you learn.

The process began with the psychiatric history, giving the psychiatrist a clear understanding of developmental and experiential elements both visible and hidden, the tripwires and reasons the patient was mired in disturbingly repetitive behaviors.

"Okay," you might say, "then why not just explain it all to the patient, so he can have an Ah-ha! moment and leave the office a new man?" The answer is: because the patient's emotional system has accumulated powerful defenses against knowing. Many defenses are helpful, but some are the source of trouble. The unconscious part of one's emotional system guards against intrusion, and if the way is not properly prepared, the patient will either brush off insights, or if presented in an unprotected moment, recoil from the exposure in anger or despair.

The process of gaining insight involves peeling back the defensive layers, revealing the part each has played in generating and preserving the individual's symptoms. It is counterintuitive: the unconscious part of our emotional system rejects unwanted, potentially discomforting new information. Meanwhile, the patient continues to deploy unconsciously-driven, often self-destructive behaviors in vain anticipation that this time things will work. *It worked when I was six; it should work again now.*

Once revealed, once the pain of exposure is endured, the patient is freed to work through the compulsion in an adaptive way, with the self—the "ego"—finally in control.

Treatment involved seeing the patient two or three times a week for a long time. Typically, analysis lasted five or more years. The more interactive "dynamic" variant typically shortened the process by half. Today, that seems absurd, and as history shows, other therapies have largely taken their place.

Our third year was almost entirely devoted to a small clutch of patients, each case supervised by a senior analyst in an hourly ratio of about three hours of therapy to one of supervision. We took meticulous notes, every word examined, especially anything we might have said to the patient. *Why did you say that? Where were you going?*

Aside from the technical aspects of treatment, there was another enormously important component in supervision: the issues of *transference* and *counter-transference*. Transference is a ubiquitous, invisible force by which previous experience is projected onto current experience and interactions. Counter-transference is a danger lurking in any treatment situation, the risk the therapist may unconsciously react to the patient's issues with his own unresolved conflicts. That is the core reason for a psychiatrist to undertake analysis. You can't treat people in depth without understanding your own psyche; otherwise, contamination with your issues is inevitable. Analysis helps keep the focus, sharpen your carefully chosen words, keeping attention entirely on the patient's problems, not yours.

My supervisors were all analysts or analysts in training. Training, incidentally, meant that a personal analysis had been completed, and a second analysis called a "training analysis" had been undertaken with a training analyst. Frankly, as I peered into the murky upper reaches of analytic work, "analysis" seemed to become a perpetual endeavor, a school of thought from which few ever seem to graduate.

As residency progressed, we did meet and present cases to some of the great gurus, cerebral rock stars of the day, all now entirely forgotten. Presentations were often in large, formal settings, well attended, scary moments, especially when the guest would pepper a resident with questions or, worse, make a withering remark about something in the presentation. I confess to one such experience.

Margaret Mahler (1897–1995), famous pediatrician, child psychiatrist, and analytic theorist, arrived with great fanfare to discuss a case in front of an audience of 400 mental health professionals anxious to hear her discuss her theories on childhood ego development. I was to present and discuss my understanding of the case. Everything was going along just fine, the end in sight as Dr. Mahler fielded one last question from the floor. Instead of answering it, she turned to me and said I should take a crack at it. It was an electron microscope moment, but I was ready, and gave what I thought to be a reasonable answer. Let's quit and go have coffee.

It was not to be. Saying she wanted to add something to my answer, she started by looking at me and saying, "There's something you don't know about the unconscious…" It was a bit like saying to a chef at the Waldorf Astoria, "There's something you don't understand about butter." I didn't hear the rest of it, and while my colleagues dismissed it entirely, I felt crushed.

Of course, I took it straightaway to the analytic couch, immediate fodder for memories of childhood humiliation, like the time my father told me, "You don't have the brains God gave a brick." Later, Dr. Mahler's research came under fire from critics who felt she got parts of her theory all wrong. *Ha! I knew it!*

Among the many gurus we encountered, there was one who stood out, a man we heard about from the start, a ghostly figure, more legend than reality. Dr. Harold Searles (1918–2015) was supposedly on the faculty, but in two-and-a-half years, the only time I had seen him was at a Christmas party. He was said to have a mystical ability to catch people—colleagues and patients alike—off guard with sudden, penetrating remarks, verbal assaults that were socially rude and professionally bad technique. Even so, his bizarre ripostes were alleged to contain pearls of extraordinary wisdom. It seemed our promised moments with the Great Man would never materialize, but late in our last year, he suddenly showed up. No warning, no announcement—he simply walked into a meeting of six of us discussing a case.

"I am Dr. Searles," he said and took a seat. He didn't ask us to introduce ourselves but flicked his wrist and casually said, "Present the case for me." It was Phil Lorio's case, and he bravely started right into his work with the difficult Mr. Gray, a man said to be no more colorful than his name. Searles listened, arms folded, nodding occasionally, and when Phil finished, he said he would like to interview the patient.

When Mr. Gray arrived, Dr. Searles introduced himself, shook the man's hand, and invited him to talk about the problems that brought him into treatment. Standard fare. No fireworks. The interview went along in what seemed like slow motion. Mr. Gray spoke in a quiet monotone, his speech unembellished, and quite frankly, boring as hell. Dr. Searles didn't seem to notice or care. He asked the occasional question, but otherwise the process droned on aimlessly for a solid thirty minutes. I was half asleep, thinking this to have been the single biggest disappointment of the entire year.

Then, with Mr. Gray in mid-sentence, Searles pounced. In a loud growling voice he said, "You know, Mr. Gray, I have a

tremendous urge to punch you in the mouth!" He paused, then
added in a quieter voice, "But I have better sense than to do it."

Oh, shit! I thought coming out of my stupor. *Where the hell
did that come from? Hang on, you're about to see a man implode right
in front of your eyes.*

It didn't happen that way. Mr. Gray sat bolt upright in his chair,
fixed his eyes on Dr. Searles, raised both hands, open palmed as if
he was about to catch a basketball, and said in a startlingly loud
voice, "YES! That's how I seem to affect lots of people!!"

Everything changed in that moment, and for another half
hour, patient and doctor had an animated conversation about Mr.
Gray's feeling permanently trapped in a windowless room. At the
end, they shook hands like old friends; Dr. Searles encouraged
him to keep working with Dr. Lorio and get busy telling people
more about how he really feels.

We were stunned, but it turned out to be a pretty normal
Searles event, based—I later realized—on the fact his understanding of the unconscious was so profound he had long since
moved beyond the world of analysis into a place where he
could comfortably grasp the deepest workings of even the most
regressed mind. From there, he felt comfortable exploring that
world with the patient without any concern about how it might
look to anyone else.

Searles' journey followed the most unlikely path, doing what
was widely considered impossible: psychoanalysis with schizophrenic patients. He would see severely regressed patients who
had been hospitalized for years, incapable of even rudimentary
conversation much less form any recognizable therapeutic relationship. He saw patients in standard fifty-minute sessions six days a
week, literally for years on end, silently enduring behavior from
profound mutism to florid psychosis.

In the only other teaching moment we had with him, Dr.
Searles described what that seemingly endless, apparently pointless process was like. By illustration, he described a woman who
for years had not spoken, but whose behavior was repetitive and

far too graphic for me to describe. It went on and on in total silence. Then one day, as he entered the room, she said, "Good morning, Dr. Searles." Recalling the moment, Searles smiled, looked up at the ceiling, and said, 'Now, *that* was a therapeutic moment."

That's about as far as he went with any explanation of his method. But behind what he said, his writing showed several key convictions. First, through his work, he had come to believe severely impaired people, especially schizophrenics, want in their depths to get better but feel disconnected with no ability to communicate with the outside world. That led him to feel that his own deeply held conflicts were a possible way to bridge the divide. So instead of taking the standard view of countertransference that saw it as a danger to be neutralized, he saw it as a tool, a way—if timed right—to reach into that void to make contact with even the most regressed patient. Look what happened with Mr. Gray: the unthinkable statement was tempered by the assurance his impulse was controlled. It was an invitation, not a threat.

Teaching encounters with luminaries like Mahler and Searles seem quaint by today's standards, but they highlight an important ingredient that over the years has seeped out of physician training in all specialties: sustained exposure to dedicated teachers. As insurance and other fiscal restraints tightened their grip in the 1970s, it became harder for programs to afford to pay highly trained, in-demand specialists. Departments once staffed by permanent faculty saw their budgets slashed, forcing faculty members into practice in order to maintain their income. Many continued to volunteer, but their work was intermittent and abbreviated, depriving trainees of precious knowledge, insights, and memorable learning experience.

Over the years, instruction time has diminished, full-time professors are a rarity, and the computer has taken over the role of teacher. With a computer at the bedside, the think-on-your feet benefit of quizzing and rapid interaction are gone, and while it is a good record keeper, and source of diagnostic coding to support billing, it is powerless to teach interactive skills, timing, and most important of all: judgment.

Behind it all is the dominant force of money. Nothing gets ahead of money, not teaching, not learning, not manners or the art of medicine. No! It's about the mighty dollar, and today's residents don't even notice it. It's just the way it is and will continue with them into practice after training is complete.

For us, money wasn't even on the table as an issue. We simply assumed we would find our way into the profession and earn a living. True, as my final year of residency was coming to an end, I did pay attention to where and how I would practice, but first 1 had one more major task to complete: present a research paper on some aspect of analytic psychiatry to the entire department, a chance showcasing our learning experience.

By that point in my training, I was thoroughly convinced the analytic approach to mental health care was far too limited to survive. It ignored too much emerging science, especially in its unhealthy resistance to the use of medication in all but the most severe cases. My parting shot was a paper on Brief Therapy, an idea starting to gain traction, a way to shape the principles of dynamic therapy into a more interactive and foreshortened format. The idea gained speed in the early 1970s, seeding a number of innovative treatment models including Interpersonal Therapy, Cognitive Therapy, and beyond.

But in July 1970, when I planned to give my talk, the idea was regarded as heretical. When the Chairman found out what I was up to, he scheduled my presentation in a small room, attended by only a handful of faculty and residents. Message received.

As I was headed out the door on my last day of residency, the Chairman shook my hand and said, "I worry about you, Phil. I hope I won't hear that you're prescribing that damn drug, lithium. It's poison." He did, however, toss me a plum by inviting me to join the Georgetown faculty to teach third- and fourth-year medical students, as well as interview residency candidates. He also asked me to run the emergency services program at DC General Hospital. I accepted both, the emergency services job for the money, the medical school job for exposure; after all, I was about to start a private practice, and I needed referrals.

This time when I got in my car, I was driving away from my last training experience. I was finally on my own, and more than a little apprehensive. It was a Tuesday, and I had exactly one new patient scheduled in the next three days. Two others were patients I had been seeing in the program and would continue to see pro bono until our work was completed. My analysis was also not finished, though at around the five-year mark, the work was terminated. When we shook hands at the door of his office, my analyst said, "Good luck. And by the way: you could have done more with dreams."

7

LOOSE ENDS

A NEWLY-MINTED RESIDENT TODAY WILL not have to go hat-in-hand begging for a job. Well ahead of graduation, she will have been recruited into a group practice, hospital, or public health staff position. Salary, compensation, work hours, vacation, and insurance will have been settled before she walks in the door. Here's your office; do you like the rug?

She certainly wouldn't be starting a solo practice in any specialty. Solo practice is nearly dead, a relic, survivable only under hybrid circumstances, such as having a spouse actively involved in managing the office. Even so, the task of keeping up with insurance billing and rejections, maintaining records, correspondence, coping with changing software issues, and lots more is exhausting and financially impossible. Yes, some brave family practitioners in rural settings manage it, but for most part, the only real answer is group, clinic, or hospital practice.

Our pathway to practice was not remotely similar to today's model. For starters, recruitments were rare; the job of finding a practice niche was entirely up to the physician. For me, it started with renting an office—a few hundred square feet, office and waiting room—bathroom down the hall. Then I sent out a printed announcement to area physicians and hospitals followed by a call to each asking for a face-to-face meeting to introduce myself. I made dozens of such calls over the next couple of months, the chance to meet and introduce myself in person. Most of the doctors were responsive, welcoming me to the physician community. It was all quite collegial, resulting in an increasing stream of referrals as well as some lasting friendships.

Growing a practice was a slow process; happily, I was able to rely on my emergency services paying job at DC General. It was basically my old job with added administrative duty, plus taking night call when one of the dozen or so psychiatrists on the panel couldn't work. That salary kept me going in the beginning.

One advantage of my porous schedule and emergency job was the opportunity to use the neurology service at DC General for board preparation. It would get me thrown in medical jail today, but in the day, not only did no one object, but the nurses and physicians were happy to help me by making charts and patients available whenever I showed up. I did tell patients I was there as part of my training, that if they were uncomfortable I would leave, but it never happened.

The service was rich in varied, sometimes obscure diseases and disorders. A similar service in an upscale hospital like Georgetown (where I was also welcome) was dull by comparison. There were plenty of stroke, seizure, and multiple sclerosis cases, but few of the more obscure, challenging syndromes likely to show up on tests.

My routine was to select a chart at random, interview the patient, do a neurological exam, then review the chart to see if my observations and conclusions matched the clinician's diagnosis. One of my favorite cases involved a very talkative man who literally hailed me as I was walking through an eight-bed room looking for a patient I had been told had a possible brain tumor. Accepting the gregarious fellow's invitation, I pulled up a chair and closed the curtain around the bed—a tight squeeze because the distance between the beds was only a few feet.

Beyond being verbal, the patient was fairly loud, overwhelming my best efforts to preserve the illusion of privacy. I plowed ahead, starting with questions about his problem, something he described in vague terms variously as a limp, headaches, and aggravation of an old injury of some sort. I weaved some cognitive status questions into the narrative, starting with "orientation;" that is, do you know who you are, where you are, and what the date is? These are questions to be repeated several times if there is even a hint of fuzzy cognition.

The patient nailed the first two, though he wasn't entirely on target with the hospital location part. But when we got to the date (it was August 1970), he said it was April 1932. *Not quite sure what day; you know, you lose time in a hospital.* Undaunted, he immediately launched into a chat about what he was doing, and how the date fit in with his activities. Later on, I came back to the question of date, to which he replied, that yes, indeed, he did know: it was January 1944, *no doubt about it,* and he took off from there on another aimless trail delivered with a sense of certainty. At the end of the interview, I asked again about the date, and without hesitation, he said it was May 1956.

With that, the man in the adjacent bed to my left, pulled back the curtain, propped up on his left elbow, and snarled at the man, "Well! You finally got it!!"

The man to the left was emerging from DTs, itself a great disrupter of memory. My patient was suffering from Korsakov's Syndrome, a disorder of memory teetering between being reversible and falling off into unchanging dementia. The most dramatic aspect of Korsakov's is *confabulation*: unconsciously made-up lies neatly patched over memory blanks, non-stop chatter presented with all the fluidity and certainty of an almost normal conversation. It is dramatic, and would be entertaining were it not such a serious condition. Its causes are many, but most commonly, the end stage of severe alcohol dependency. The man with DTs would likely recover, had a better chance of regaining cognitive functioning, perhaps even using it to stay sober before another, possibly fatal, withdrawal crisis. The outlook for the Korsakov's patient was bleak.

I also started to teach in the medical school—no salary, but more exposure, plus it was fun. At least it started off as fun. Just as I had experienced psychiatry in medical school with less than full attention, so, too, in spite of my best efforts, my students listened in glassy-eyed indifference. It's different when you're on the other side of the lectern. *Hey! Don't ignore this! It's important!* It was like shoveling fleas.

In my second year of teaching, it got dramatically worse when I was confronted with a particularly defiant student. He was a senior without the faintest interest in anything I had to say. He was going to graduate in the spring anyway, and nothing I said seemed to penetrate. When he went from yawning apathy to skipping class, I warned him of the consequences. When he skipped the midyear exam, I went to the dean to express my alarm, but he just shrugged, told me to give him a remake and stop worrying. It took three attempts before he finally took the test. He failed. With graduation approaching, he simply stopped coming at all. Several trips to the dean's office netted nothing. He skipped the final, so I turned in a failing grade, fully aware that it would derail his graduation. The dean hit the roof, told me to give him a remake, and when I argued the point, the dean said *he* would give the remake, I was off the hook. No surprise, he passed and graduated on time. A month later, I received a thank you note expressing gratitude for my work but saying my services were no longer needed.

My next disappointment was the collapse of the emergency services job. Sadly, it was largely over a turf and race issue. DC General was overwhelmingly African American in both patients and staff. The emergency services unit, however, was staffed almost exclusively with white psychiatrists. There was a lot of pressure to change that, but efforts to hire more African American psychiatrists were halting at best. As frustration grew, so did hostility. The panel was collapsing, and I realized it would be best to leave the position.

That was the end of my access to DC General; fortunately, by that time, I was shifting away from neurology back toward board preparation focused increasingly on medication and brain chemistry as we knew it—almost primitive by today's standards.

The written boards were long and tedious, but the orals were an entirely different matter. I was able to take the written part in

Washington, DC, but a year later, I had to go to Chicago to take the orals. That trip was thoroughly enjoyable, the cases carefully selected, and the examiners were more teachers than inquisitors.

By far the best moment was when I was examining a neurology patient at the Chicago VA Hospital. The examiner wanted to observe my examination technique, not go through a diagnostic interview. Better, of course, if I picked up abnormalities that could suggest a diagnosis. At the end, he asked me to list possible diagnoses suggested by the examination itself—then take a stab at the diagnosis.

The patient had clearly been through this before, knew exactly what I was up to, and seemed to enjoy the experience. As I was looking at his retina, my ears only inches from his mouth, he whispered, "Weak as a kitten. Inherited. Bet you haven't seen this one before." I noted a fresh scar on his arm, asked *sotto voce* if it was a biopsy. "Yes," he whispered.

Obviously, he had an unusual muscle disease, not a more routine dystrophy, a condition that didn't readily give itself away. There are a host of muscle diseases I had never seen before, though at least I had something to go on, thanks to the patient. When it came to diagnosis, I said what I knew: that it was a rare, probably heritable dystrophy, adding that a muscle biopsy would likely tell the tale. I said I didn't know what disease he had and did my best to list all the oddball diseases I could think of, including McArdle Disease. The examiner seemed satisfied, told me it was indeed McArdle Disease, and spent the rest of our time teaching me some of the finer points of diagnosing dystrophies.

By that time—three years into practice—it was becoming increasingly clear that the days of reliance on classical psychotherapy were numbered. Insurance was tightening up, and pressure to prescribe was building. Antidepressant and antipsychotic drugs were still loaded with side effects, not exactly "poison," to use the residency director's descriptor, but potentially dangerous if not used with selective caution.

A decade later, in the late 1980s, Prozac hit the market, followed by a flood of new drugs, all touted as less toxic and more effective than the old ones. While they were certainly easier to tolerate, they were not without side effects, especially metabolic dangers. In spite of industry propaganda, they did not appear to be more effective than the older drugs, but because they had fewer initial side effects, patients were more willing to stick with them long enough to show results.

The issue of long-term side effects was unknown and largely ignored by manufacturers, a repeating pattern with virtually all new drugs. Because the initial number taking them is low, only the most obvious side effects are seen, and many of them are not side effects at all. Things like dry mouth and upset stomach are all *direct effects* of the drug, relatively benign, the *expected* response to introducing a new chemical into the body. The line between direct and side effects is fuzzy, but generally, direct effects are more annoying than dangerous, while true side effects are unexpected, ranging from troublesome to catastrophic.

Exactly the same pattern followed the introduction of novel antipsychotic drugs in the 1990s, initially ballyhooed as both easier to take and more effective than antiques from a decade before. What can possibly go wrong? Plenty, as it happens. The moral is always the same: enthusiastic acceptance of the glories of new medication is a fool's game.

Sadly, as we moved out of the 1990s, "Medication Management" increasingly took over as the forced model for psychiatric care. Similar pressure existed in other specialties, but not as profoundly as in psychiatry. The large mental health clinic where I worked had nearly 500 employees, mostly administrative, but only a handful of psychiatrists. Office managers dictated increasing constriction of our time with patients, pushing speed over quality, always bleating about productivity.

The medical model of care was challenged, often to the point of absurdity. I was constantly in hot water for refusing to call patients "clients" or worse, "customers," and criticizing the administration's preoccupation with meaningless ethics and management training. Near the end, when I told the director I had studied the matter and realized the *real* problem with ethics lay with the agency's inability to offer meaningful psychiatric services, I was told to put it in writing—a surefire preamble to getting me fired.

Fortunately for me, I was on the verge of retirement and left before I could be canned. When I drove away that afternoon, it was the only time since graduating from medical school 48 years before that I wasn't headed for another assignment. I went home, had a drink, and the next day, notified the state licensing bureau that I had retired and would no longer need to renew my license. It wasn't a petulant or bitter move; it simply meant I was quite happy to be ending that phase of my life, grateful for the experience, and ready for the next challenge.

I also started to write down reflections on my experience, the start of this book. Having stepped away from the career, I was able to look back, free to review what was suddenly becoming history. But since retiring, a number of trends in training and practice seem to have accelerated dramatically and demand some additional attention, including risking some thoughts about the current national debate about the delivery of health care.

Fifty years ago, the message was "Medicine's great tradition is in your hands. Take what you know and continue to learn to practice with honor and skill." The government was largely invisible, insurance was helpful, Pharma was focused on research, medications were affordable, gaming the system from within was a rarity, and technology was carrying our noble profession forward.

Certainly, technology continues to fulfill its mission, all the way from computers and CT scans to robotic surgery, yet even progress has its price. Technological advances are helpful and cost effective when carefully applied to answer clinical questions or conduct screening for disease. Overenthusiasm, however, is hugely expensive, unnecessary, and even dangerous. Just because we *can* doesn't mean we *should*.

Mammography, prostate testing, routine ultrasound, CT imaging tests, and more may look like prudence in every case, but they are not surefire, to say nothing of the hair-raising and expensive consequences of false positives. The worst of the lot is the full body scan, hardly ever uncovering a symptomless, deadly intruder lurking at the gate. But, brother, can it find the "maybe" problems! Then what? Chase every shadow? Go after every little spot with a biopsy needle? Or tell the anxious patient, "We'll watch it," with another study in six months.

But the CYA (cover your ass) factor is huge. No one sues because you were too cautious. The worst that can happen is the charge is rejected by the insurance carrier, and the unfortunate patient is stuck with the entire bill. Lost in all of this is the time-honored recognition that most diseases send a symptom signal, one that an alert patient working with a careful physician can find and treat. But *reasonable* has given way to *absolute*, especially if someone else is footing the bill.

A perfect example of the cost of misdirected thinking and dollars is the way we mistreat elderly patients in their last moments of life. Medicare squanders bails of money tormenting dying patients with painful tests and futile treatments instead of helping patient and family accept the reality of imminent death, easing rather than complicating the process. The cost is staggering: nearly 30% of Medicare's budget is spent on patients in their last six months of life, a goodly portion in the final days.

Just bringing up the idea of changing our end-of-life behavior causes apoplexy among people who instantly assume it to be code for euthanasia. Just the suggestion that physicians have a frank discussion with the patient and family prompts some to cry, "Death Squads!" Others fear it implies rationing care in people with terminal illness just to save money. None of it could be farther from the truth. It is simply about stepping back to rethink the way we currently handle care of people in their last moments of life. If pre-death heroics saved lives or provided relief from pain, it would be worth it. But they simply do not.

Consider: Do you want to end up in the ICU with tubes in every orifice while your family paces the hallway hoping for a miracle that won't happen? Or would you prefer hospice care in a peaceful, dignified, and comfortable setting for both you and your family, with "treatment" focused on providing the right amount of medication to maintain comfort? Like so many aspects of our derailed system, ideological misdirection quickly becomes political, preventing thoughtful debate, and preserving the status quo.

Something has also gone profoundly wrong within the medical profession itself. My colleagues are almost universally discouraged, find practice tedious, seeing themselves as nothing more than pawns in a vast financial game. I have yet to meet a single one who would do it over again, or recommend a career in medicine. They all say the same thing: who wants to start with a mountain of debt, the uncertainty of practice opportunity, ending up just another cog in the corporate wheel, or a salaried employee in a government-run system?

Virtually every time I visit or interact socially with an older physician, I hear the same refrain: *Boy! Are you lucky you're retired! I can't wait!* One PCP told me a decade ago, *"I'd rather pump gas."* It's harder to hear what the younger ones think, especially in an office setting. You're lucky to have a few minutes to present your problem. Small talk with the ancients is not wanted.

There is, however, a slowly spreading national apprehension about health care, though it is still mired in slogans and opinions flying about without a clear idea of what's wrong, much less what a fix would look like.

Let's start with the basics. As a nation we spend far more per capita on health care than any other nation, around 17% of GDP, 25% more than second place Switzerland and Norway, yet we rank 11th among wealthy nations in quality and access to health care. We do a dismal job with prevention, have fewer doctors and nurses, and fewer graduating physicians per capita compared to other wealthy nations. Particularly alarming, access to primary care and appointment speed are well down the ranking scale.

We certainly do a lot of things well, including stroke care, management of heart attack, controlling hospital infection, and detection of colorectal, breast, and cervical cancer. But hospital costs are through the ceiling, and the use of emergency rooms for routine care is well above average, largely because of lack of insurance and access to primary care.

Beyond statistics, it is inescapably clear that in spite of the widely held perception we have the best health care in the world, we simply do not. It's good, but it is frightfully expensive and inefficient. Other nations have simplified systems. Not us. We have multiple, competing systems, each with its own structure and rules. Access and quality of care are weighted toward those in programs like Medicare, Medicaid, the Veteran's system, employer-supported insurance, or who simply have the money to pay out of pocket no matter what the cost. The rest are at the mercy of the brainless marketplace. Will Rogers said, "'Em as has, gits." Nowhere is that more true than in access to healthcare today.

The number of people currently without any sort of health insurance is around 27 million; equally alarming, the number of people with inadequate health care is over 30 million—and rising. Even with a basic health insurance plan, a simple hospital stay or ER visit can result in crushing expense. Two thirds of all bankruptcies in the US—over 500 thousand a year—result from medical debt.

Since the early 1970s, the driving force behind medical training and clinical practice has been increasing preoccupation with money. Marketplace economics have saturated every aspect of health care delivery, a force with no soul, and just one goal: profit. As a country, we value free enterprise and reject any suggestion of controlling markets. We equate competition with efficiency, overlook abuse within the system, and see the resulting concentration of wealth, power, and control as entirely benign.

Medicine has become corporatized right under our noses, its needs nurtured by a submissive congress guided by industry lobbyists. A senator who dares support consumer-friendly legislation risks being crushed in an avalanche of pushback, loss of campaign funding, and the threat of being sent home to practice law in a second-floor office with no heat.

Before you conclude this to be a preamble to a plea for a single payer solution, it is not. We can't talk about solutions until we grasp the problem, starting with agreement that the system is broken and must be fixed. Stir in some historical perspective plus facts we can actually agree on, and then we may be able to arrive at something approaching a consensus. Naïve? Perhaps, but the default position is argument with slogans and bumper stickers, financed by players convinced they already have the answers. Vote for me!

Remember the early 1990s when the Clintons tried to introduce a single payer system? It failed miserably, undermined because the country was not on board. It came out of nowhere, was complex, backlash was resounding, and—predictably—it all fell apart. The same thing will happen again without an informed electorate thinking about what may be wrong, ready for clear-headed consideration of our options.

Resistance comes mainly from three sources, starting with health care corporations who own hospitals, clinical practices (like the one your PCP is in), nursing homes, and medical equipment and pharmacy chains, entities that used to operate individually, just happy to serve and stay in the black. Then there are myriad insurance companies diverting an enormous amount of money away from health care into the pockets of shareholders, investors, and excessively compensated executives. By contrast, single payer administrations spend far less money on salaries, non-medical compensation, and advertising. "Well," you say, "we don't have that sort of socialist nonsense in our country!" Yes, we do: Medicare, Medicaid, and the VA are all single payer systems—and they're popular. In fact, the VA system is actually a form of socialized medicine because the system owns the facilities, pays the salaries, and controls the cost of drugs. It's only the insured, underinsured, and uninsured who live in the marketplace.

The third group is Pharma, every bit as voracious as the others. Pharma has fattened itself on lax rules, Part D government protection, advertising, and the seemingly innocuous effort to better classify and define disease and related disorders.

The "better classification" story is pretty dry cereal but hugely important in understanding how the financial system took advantage of science. In a nutshell: as medical insurance, Medicare, Medicaid, and the VA all gathered steam in the 1970s, pressure mounted to define and classify diseases and treatment procedures with precision, written in universally accepted codes. As high-minded as the effort was, it had the secondary effect of expanding the way we define disease. If five major and three lesser criteria were needed to diagnose a disease, it followed that having two of each must mean the patient *almost* has it. That called for the invention of the *spectrum concept* with new names for diagnosis-lite disturbances. It didn't take long for that to spill over into the edges of normal behavior, making almost anything treatable, and more to the point: billable.

Pharma responded with new drugs, not just in psychiatry, but in all specialties. As the idea of treating more people grew, companies often got around FDA rules on exactly how a given drug could be prescribed by going "off label." For example, if a drug approved for treating psychosis also has a potent effect on sleep, then why not give a wee dose to your insomnia patients? Even when Pharma was caught and fined, the practice continued. The money rolled in. Incidentally, going off label is allowed when the physician documents both the rationale behind its use and the fact it has been fully explained to the patient. Ever had that chat with your doctor? I doubt it.

But until 1997, Pharma couldn't advertise directly to consumers, so they did the next best thing: market their products to physicians using bribery disguised as a selfless combination of education and practice support. While grandly costumed to disguise their intent, it all came down to flattery and money dispensed by an army of seducers steering physicians into favoring their products.

Their tools were many, including paid vacation seminars, meetings pretending to probe physicians for suggestions and feedback on their drugs, as well as lucrative positions on their speaker panels. Typically, the well-paid Trojan speaker presented a pseudo-neutral discussion at a lavish dinner, a talk that somehow always managed to highlight the glories of the sponsor's product while basically ignoring the rival's product.

Pharmaceutical "reps," as they were called, visited one's office with free samples, scientific papers favoring their product, coffee cups, paperweights, pens, and sandwiches for the entire staff. The reps were themselves well compensated, affable, and skillful in touting their wares. Among the many reps I have known, two stand out as the most perfect example of exactly how corrupt the system is.

I'll call them Bob and Ray, friends representing the same pharmaceutical company, covering several large towns in a mostly rural state. Nothing strange about it on the surface, but underneath, a huge tug of war was taking place focused almost exclusively on two rival practices. The two physicians running those practices openly disliked each other and competed aggressively for business. More importantly from the drug company's perspective, they dispensed an enormous amount of the company's medications, well over one million dollars' worth a year of one medication alone.

Because of the caustic dynamics and massive revenue streams, the company assigned Bob to one practice, Ray to the other. The two men had to pretend loyalty, including never being seen together socially. If a dinner presentation was anticipated to hype a product, there had to be two identical dinners with separate audiences. The entire medical community was divided, like fans at a soccer match there to cheer on their man.

In a candid moment, reflecting on the absurdity of the situation, Bob told me, "Put it this way: if my guy calls at two o'clock in the morning to tell me he wants his porch painted, I'd be there in an hour."

I don't want to sound too holy about this because in the beginning I was very much a part of it. Dr. Just-Finished-His-Analysis slipped right in-line, accepted the trips to La Costa and Disney World, became a frequent speaker, and had no trouble cashing the checks. The breaking point came when one of the companies invited me to join a small, "exclusive" group for a meeting at Headquarters, the ultimate reward for all of my hard work on behalf of patients. Translation: all the hard work you do writing prescriptions for our products.

The "big moment" came when we were invited to go into the Board of Directors Conference Room, take a seat around the table—*one sugar or two?*—while the CEO lavished praise on our work. It was one flattery too far. And when I shared my experience with some colleagues, I quickly became aware that there had been a steady parade of "exclusive" groups sequenced through the "Halls of Flattery." Snap. That was it. Funny, but once you see it, you can't imagine how you let yourself get snagged in the first place.

The entire effort came under increasing fire in the 1990s, but no matter, the industry was getting a brand-new tool, one that made the clumsy business of arranging all those trips to Ocean World obsolete. Cut out the middleman! Go straight to the market's core: *advertise directly to the consumer!*

Direct advertising to consumers is less about law than the regulatory authority of the FDA (Food and Drug Administration). When I was in training, samples flowed freely, including amphetamines, barbiturates, pain pills, and more. I was given a few basics like a medical bag, but that was about it. Detail reps were relatively few, not the least pushy, and quite helpful with literature searches on virtually any subject. In 1969 the FDA put restrictions on direct advertising by requiring clear disclosure of side effects and contraindications. In the seventies well into the eighties advertising was predominantly directed at doctors, mostly through reps and printed media. Some changes were made in the mid-eighties, but the dam held pretty well until 1997 when the FDA weakened disclosure requirements seen by industry to be too burdensome.

That did it. No more wasting money on coffee cups, time to go to the heart of the matter, invest some real money, and stop pretending everything is about education and patient welfare. Screw that. Use the print media to tell patients what they need, and let's see how well the doctors stand up to that kind of pressure! Since then, the money spent on advertising has soared—along with profits. The onslaught has been massive and highly effective.

The United States and New Zealand are the only two countries in the world that allow direct advertising to consumers.

Currently, all but one of the top ten drug companies spend more on advertising than on R&D (research and development), some by a wide margin. So much for the argument they need high prices to support R&D.

There is another danger hidden in the money cloud: advertising drugs is only as effective as the number of patients buying them. Operating hand-in-glove with the expansion of advertising is the good news about enthusiasm for expanded diagnosis beyond the limits of outdated concepts. It is no coincidence that the number of kids said to have ADHD has soared. So, too, the number of depressed people said to need all those antidepressants. Bipolar Disorder? Once a complex diagnosis with crisp borders, it is now up for grabs with any combination of irritability and dysphoria on the patient's side, added to time and patient pressure on the doctor's side.

A story illustrates the point.

In the early 2000s, I treated a young woman struggling to make ends meet, burdened by some bad interpersonal decisions, but determined to push her way through to something better. She had some episodic, low-level depression, some realistic anxiety, but happily she never used drugs, and worked whenever she could find a job that paid enough to cover childcare. I saw her regularly for several years, always impressed by her determination and dedication to her kids.

Five or six years later, I met her on the street, and asked how she was doing. I noticed she had gained a significant amount of weight, and immediately began to suspect medication was the cause, though for obvious reasons, I didn't ask anything about her treatment. She immediately told me she had a new psychiatrist who realized her *real* problem was Bipolar Disorder and started her on "the right medications" (plural), as well as helping her get SSDI disability. When I knew her, there had been no indication of bipolarity in her history or symptoms; worse, the powerhouse drugs she was taking were making her a metabolic ruin. I wished her well. I'll bet my hat she's diabetic today.

Diagnostic and treatment inflation are not limited to psychiatry: they cross the board in every specialty. Going bald, maybe a little bit? Use this! Sex life not what you imagine it should be? You probably have a disorder called ED (erectile dysfunction). Take one of these drugs, look at the world through a heart pounding new blue light. In this category of expansion (no pun intended), the line between *disease* and *desire* gets fuzzy. The number of people with clearly defined, medically-induced ED isn't even closely matched with the number of people seeking the medication. Once started, the "patient" is reluctant to stop. *Maybe I won't be able to perform as well!*

Perhaps the biggest co-expansion of all of diagnosis and treatment—certainly the most catastrophic—is the monster called pain management. Pressure to prescribe pain medication shortcuts access to the myriad other, non-medication interventions such as improved nutrition, exercise, physical therapy, treatment of comorbid conditions, and psychotherapy. Applied individually or together, actual control of pain is possible. Pain medications by themselves simply don't work. They don't *treat* pain, they hardly control it, and are fraught with side effects including habituation and addiction. Insulin controls blood sugar, thyroid hormone controls some forms of thyroid disease, and chemotherapy can cure cancer. But pain meds? Great for profits, but prolonged use is terrible—even deadly—for patients.

Kids with bad temper problems, or any of a number of other non-disease issues of childhood, are suddenly diagnosed as having a form of ADHD. How? Often through the concept of "spectrum"; again, having *some* signs of a disorder is the same as having it. The same goes for having *some* symptoms of depression, *some* symptoms associated with autism, *some* variation of migraine, or any number of repetitive behaviors suddenly labeled as *addiction*.

Hard-pressed PCPs are pushed into prescribing for ADHD, anxiety, and depressive disorders. Access to specialists is slow and cumbersome, especially for child psychiatry. It's simply easier to prescribe the drugs. Or if the patient has been seen and diagnosed by a specialist in any field, the patient may be returned to the PCP with the expectation he will continue the medication program without a clear plan of when and how to modify or stop treatment.

I imagine a two-frame cartoon in the *New Yorker*:

First frame: Two friends meet on the street, one looking downtrodden.

"Why so gloomy, Fred? Are you sick?" one asks.

"My doctor did a bunch of tests and said I'm okay."

"Bummer!" replies his friend.

Second frame: They meet again on the street, this time the patient looks cheerful.

"You look better, Fred!"

"Yeah. My doctor gave me some medicine—just in case."

"Great! Now you're getting somewhere!"

Diagnostic plasticity and expanded drug use have also affected the disability scene. Like my former patient newly diagnosed as bipolar, many more are applying for and getting disability. Attempts to tighten criteria have generally failed over lack of agreement about how to define and apply diagnostic criteria.

So, what's the answer? We've looked at some of the problems, where do we go from here?

Any good plan starts with clear goals a proposed solution must achieve. Since a nation can only be as productive as its citizens are healthy, and since the cost of health care drops as people's health improves, it stands to reason we should be focused on providing everyone with access to quality health care. Easy so far, but to work, achieving access must also be affordable. Now it's getting sticky.

There is no free lunch, and like it or not, we have to deal with two related problems: rationing and paying for system upgrades.

We already ration access, hiding that reality in copays, deductibles, restrictions on preexisting conditions, high premiums, drug price tiers, the donut hole, or any of a dozen other filtering mechanisms, all of them hard at work controlling costs. Let's be honest and out in the open about exactly what we are willing to pay for, and what we are not. Add *transparency* to our list of goals.

Saying "everybody" must be covered is misleading, as it implies a massive overhaul. But let's not forget that most of the population is already covered through Medicare, Medicaid, the VA, and employer-sponsored insurance. The problem area is the uninsured and underinsured. Increasing premiums or raising deductibles are out of the question for this group. Similarly, bleeding already anemic policies gets us nowhere. Mandating coverage for preexisting conditions puts further pressure on cost.

All of this takes us to the inevitable reality of some combination of market intervention and public funding; anathema to many, but unavoidable if we want to solve the problem. The Affordable Care Act increased the number of insured significantly, but attempts to do even more were stymied when the requirement that everyone in the insurance pool share the costs was scotched. The simple fact about any type of insurance is that it cannot work if only the neediest pay a premium. Curiously, Social Security *Insurance* and Medicare *Insurance* are widely accepted, both financed through taxes paid for decades before one can actually benefit from either. You can't buy homeowner's insurance the day your stove catches fire. The same for life insurance: buy it when you are young and it's cheap. Wait too long and it's prohibitively expensive—if you can get it at all.

It seems obvious that group participation combined with some type of public support is inevitable. The question is, exactly what form does that "support" take? How much messing with the marketplace is going to be needed—or tolerated?

One stumbling block is the way insurance companies fritter away oceans of money on administrative costs, salaries, and advertising. One answer is to intervene in that process.

But suggesting intervention in the vast free market insurance industry is one step too far. Even knowing about the millions of dollars wasted on generating profits, money that could be directed to benefit consumers, we tremble at the mere mention of intervening in a private sector business model. We have to get over the idea that talking about something is somehow the same as doing it.

Why not imagine ways to develop a more streamlined template for health insurance policies? Right now there are hundreds of different policies to cope with, a paperwork nightmare for every healthcare facility. Wouldn't a more universal billing system coupled with streamlined policies save a lot of money? The insurance companies are good at handling billing and payment systems. Let them continue in a more simplified system, make a profit, but tame advertising and executive compensation, and insist they live up to their own lofty promises: We commit to being our members' trusted partner in providing affordable, innovative products that improve their care and health (Blue Cross Blue Shield mission statement).

Germany has one of the best health care systems in the world, vastly less expensive and more efficient than ours. It does so through over two hundred insurance carriers managing streamlined, non-profit policies with universal requirements, including strong emphasis on prevention. Doctors bill their services for patients seen, but their fees are regulated. About 10 percent of the population opts for more expensive private insurance.

In 2010, the Affordable Care Act (ACA) was passed, mandating everyone have some form of health insurance, plans that must include coverage for preexisting conditions (previously the penultimate rationing device), support for primary care, decreased billing complexity, and increased attention to prevention. The act mandated companies spend 80 percent of their premiums on care, and took aim at the cost of drugs, including trying to close the donut hole.

Not everyone wanted to buy policies under the new law, even with devices in place to support those who could not afford the full weight of premiums. To maximize the payment pool, in 2014 the ACA's controversial "mandate" went into effect, a provision decreeing a fine be levied against those who did not buy insurance. It was hugely unpopular. Younger, healthier people didn't see why they had to be forced to buy something they didn't need; for others, it was simply a matter of opposition to government intrusion, the slippery slope to full-on control of health care.

The ACA also pressed states to increase Medicaid coverage for those on the bottom end who couldn't afford the ACA at all. In spite of federal payments to soften the expansion, many states balked. That left millions out in the cold. They had too much to get Medicaid, too little to buy even the most slimmed down policies.

The Supreme Court upheld the mandate system but knocked down the ACA requirement that states increase Medicaid coverage. The Tax Cuts and Jobs Law of 2017 eliminated the mandate, starting in 2019. Meanwhile, a number of states, seeing the looming cost of care about to fall on them, introduced their own mandates. Around 35 states accepted Medicaid expansion funds, the rest did not.

So, the battle rages. Inevitably we have to figure out if we're going to repair the current system or come up with something entirely new. We also have to decide if we are going to reform Part D to allow negotiating lower drug costs, and if some reform in end-of-life issues in Medicare can be made. Certainly, we have to invest more in prevention. Imagine the cost of obesity alone to our economy. Or turn it around: imagine the savings from even modest improvement. All of this is tough to talk about, but we cannot afford to keep dodging it.

I am not sure how much the various proposals would cost. The government now spends around $700 billion a year on subsidized programs for people under 65. That includes Medicaid, CHIP (Children's Health Insurance Program), disability entitlements, and the cost of employer write-offs for employee health plans. In its original form, ACA subsidies were going to be somewhere north of $50 billion. But in a reimagined ACA plan covering more people with fewer limitations, the numbers are harder to find, largely because any significant change would cause a reshuffling between programs like Medicaid and employer insurance. Even with savings from having a healthier nation, costs are still staggering. By contrast: we have spent about two trillion dollars on the war in Afghanistan. We throw away about $150 billion dollars' worth of food every year. We are at the bottom of comparable countries in taxation, our gas is cheap, and people scream like wounded eagles at even a hint of increased taxes on anything. We think of ourselves as the world's greatest democracy, yet we seem helpless to even begin tackling the health care problems virtually every other country has taken bold steps to correct.

The marketplace has many virtues, but willingness to accept any suggestion of change isn't one of them. It is efficient in generating technology, competition, and corporate profit, but inept when it comes to distributing benefit across the board. It produces a modest product for many, but painful indifference for far too many others. It's time to break out of our denial and start a real discussion of how to deal with an urgency bordering on a crisis. Forget slogans and seductive promises of quickie solutions. The only bumper sticker I want to see is the one that says, "The mind is like a parachute: it only works when it's open." Read, think, debate, and speak up.

Meanwhile, I've got my feet up on the porch railing, enjoying wonderful memories of good fortune that started with the summer of stolen moments divided between my grandmother's house at one end of the hollow and Granny Cleek's at the other. I see Grandmother, putter in hand, getting into her Rolls Royce. Then I see Granny, hatchet in hand, stepping into her hen house.

It was pure, undeserved luck to have started life at both ends of the road.

ACKNOWLGEMENTS

OF THE MANY PEOPLE I have to thank for helping me through my work, my wife deserves the first cheer. Writing is a self-absorbed, time-consuming process, and tolerating it takes a lot of patience and generosity of spirit. She gave up time for my research excursions and weekend writing sessions—more undeserved good fortune.

When I started this project, I made the assumption I would be able to get a grip on the current state of medical education simply by interviewing medical school faculty, students, and PGY residents. Similarly, I planned to take the pulse of medical practice by talking to colleagues and others in active practice. It turned out to be harder than I thought.

Multiple attempts to get interviews with medical school deans and teachers were either ignored or simply declined. Even a school where I had a previous faculty appointment was not interested. When I did finally get some interview time, it was brief and defensive.

The reason was simple: they all feared having something unfavorable written about their institution. So play it safe—just say "No." Defensive medicine is universal; turns out, so is administrative caution.

Students were no different, but their motivation was simpler: they really didn't care. They have no interest in talking about older teaching methods, or how we managed before the invention of the computer, scanner, or instant-read lab results. Most have their career plan laid out, loans to repay, and...*Excuse me, I've got to get to a class.*

Jerry Ringland, MD, OB-GYN practitioner, teacher, and friend, helped with late-night discussions and introductions to fellow professors, including two acknowledged experts in medical education and clinical care: Steven Bergmann, PhD, MD, with Penn Medical Center (Princeton, NJ), and William J. Ledger, MD, former Chairman of Obstetrics and Gynecology at Weill Cornell Medical College. Both were candid, thought my inquiry had merit, and shared their considerable knowledge openly—even bluntly.

Physician friends and colleagues working in independent groups were far more forthcoming in their assessment than those in corporate practice settings. The independent cohort, as one friend put it, is still allowed to "practice." The corporate folks are "managed." Many from both groups said how much they envied me being retired. The older they are, the more they want to get out. Some of the younger ones express disappointment at being contained by loans and endless rules governing their practice.

There is another small group of professionals I want to thank: medical school librarians and archivists. For the archivists, history matters. And for the librarians, there is still satisfaction in helping researchers find accurate, often obscure, information.

The day I walked into the archives at my *alma mater*, Jefferson Medical College (Thomas Jefferson University), I was stunned to see Dr. Gibbon's heart-lung machine disassembled on a large table. It turns out there was a group of researchers coming in to examine the relic. It seemed like a sign.

Among the many helpful librarians I met, one in particular stands out: Ms. Jody Coste at the Medical College of Virginia (Virginia Commonwealth University School of Medicine). She didn't need to get out a lot of books to answer many of my questions, and when she did have to search, it only took a few minutes to find the right reference. Even more important was her willingness to talk about some truly thorny questions about MCV's history, issues the deans would prefer to avoid. She readily acknowledged the inherent racism and sexism in the old system. She also had no hesitation in talking about the fact that organs were indeed harvested under shady circumstances. Nor was she surprised to hear about unacknowledged abortions or the reluctance to investigate one of the feared Dr. Hume's team members.

There are a prodigious number of books and articles available about the state of medical care, its progression over time, and problems today. The bookshelves are jammed; where to begin? A good start would be, Kenneth Ludmerer's *Time to Heal: American Medical Education from the Turn of the Century to the Era of Managed Care* (Oxford Press, 1999). For a slant on what is going on today, pick up *Saving Normal* by Allen Frances (Harper Collins Publisher, 2014). While it is focused on what has happened in the field of psychiatry, my main interest over the years, the concepts and examples apply neatly across the entire medical spectrum. His ideas on "diagnostic inflation" are particularly insightful.

No matter where you start, remember: it's your health we are talking about.

ABOUT THE AUTHOR

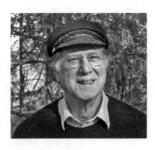 PHILIP HIRSH QUIBBLES WITH THE word "author." He prefers "writer," a reflection of his sense that he is a reporter describing what he knows and has experienced, feeling it may have value to a reader both as information, and perhaps a pathway out of the box—a new way to look at old ideas. He wants the story to speak for itself, unobscured with flowered prose. It doesn't matter if the subject is fiction or fact, nor if the speaker is a person or a horsefly, as long as the story and message are clear. *Health Care Gone Wrong* is a reporter's summary of half a century in the medical profession, talking about schools, hospitals, prisons, the army—all of it, both on and off the beaten path.

When Evil Isn't Enough was Hirsh's first novel, a test to see if he could wrap his ideas into a crime story. *Voices from the Hollow* was next, short stories about Appalachian people and their culture. It was a finalist in *Foreword* magazine's short story Book of the Year award in 2006. *The Lost Tarpon* is a collection of fanciful stories ranging from bemused to lacerating, all trying to pull the fig leaf off of conventional morality. *Surviving Justice* carries that theme into a novel about a man sent to San Quentin prison for a murder he did not commit. After 52 years, he is unexpectedly released into a world he no longer recognizes. The forces that sent him to prison years before are watching, and want him back in prison. Or even better: dead. Using his prison skills, he manages to survive—and find justice. The book is currently under contract to become a motion picture.

Dr. Hirsh was educated at Phillips Academy, Andover, Yale University and Jefferson Medical College. He is retired. He and his wife live on the eastern shore of Maryland.

CPSIA information can be obtained
at www.ICGtesting.com
Printed in the USA
FSHW021712221021
85650FS